MEDICINE WOMAN

RECLAIMING THE SOUL
OF HEALING

Lucy H. Pearce

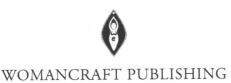

WOMANCRAFT PUBLISHING

COPYRIGHT AND DISCLAIMER

ENDORSEMENTS

This is Lucy Pearce's opus – a body of work which requires a lifetime of preparation to garner this kind of courage that boldly sets raw truth free. In doing so her words unshackle others too. Medicine Woman is a clarion call in a world where we are needing to heal generational wounds, to own where we have been complicit so we can make room for the collective rise that seeks another way forward.

ALisa Starkweather, founder of the Red Tent Temple Movement

Lucy Pearce is a luminous voice in global change – a voice that calls out for a return to balance of the feminine and masculine energies to heal the very world all beings depend upon to continue existing – preferably thriving. Medicine Woman is needed wake up words in a world gone numb.

Paula Youmell, RN, Wise Woman Nurse®, author *Hands on Health* and *Weaving Healing Wisdom*

Lucy Pearce writes with a blazing mix of passion and vulnerability as she boldly explores the complexities of health issues facing contemporary women. This hard-hitting narrative exposes the undeniable bias that shapes modern medicine and keeps women sick. Pearce gives voice to the silent epidemic of invisible illness. Her revelations are cataclysmic. With an unwavering commitment to healing, and through harnessing the primal creative power of the feminine, this book offers real hope to those who suffer. Medicine Woman heralds the reclaiming of our innate power to heal ourselves. This deeply personal work offers all women the opportunity to take full responsibility for our lives and thrive.

Teresa Maria Bilowus, woman, mother, author, mentor and founder of the 'Voices From The Red Tent' project

In Medicine Woman, Lucy H. Pearce continues her invaluable work of re-awakening the Sacred Feminine and connecting women to their inherent wisdom. Pulling back the curtain on the male-dominated medical model of the current era, Pearce reveals the systematic and intentional suppression of feminine knowledge and intuition, and in doing so invites modern women to reclaim their own healing journey. The Medicine Woman archetype is needed in our culture now more than ever as women awaken to the healing power and potential that lies within each of us.

Amy Bammel Wilding, author *Wild & Wise: Sacred Feminine Meditations for Women's Circles and Personal Awakening*

For my grandmother, Lucy Crocker Pearce,
in loving memory and gratitude for being a pioneer
in so many aspects of health and community.

For all the women, throughout the ages,
who were not treated with the compassion they deserved.

For we who are still not now,
That we may heal ourselves
And the world.

ALSO BY LUCY H. PEARCE

Books

Full Circle Health: integrated health charting for women
(Womancraft Publishing, 2017)

Full Circle Health: 3-month charting journal (Womancraft Publishing, 2017)

Burning Woman (Womancraft Publishing, 2016)

Moon Time: harness the ever-changing energy of your menstrual cycle
(Womancraft Publishing, 2015)

Reaching for the Moon: a girl's guide to her cycles (Womancraft Publishing, 2015)

Moods of Motherhood: the inner journey of mothering
(Womancraft Publishing, 2014)

The Rainbow Way: cultivating creativity in the midst of motherhood
(Soul Rocks, 2013)

E-courses – see www.lucyhpearce.com:

WORD+image   *Your Authentic Voice*

Be Your Own Publisher   *Structuring the Soul of Writing*

Contributor to:

Demystifying The Artist; The Power of Ritual; Naked Money, Eli Trier (2018)

Goddess: When She Rules: expressions by contemporary women
(Golden Dragonfly Press, 2018)

We'Moon Diary – La Luna (2018), Fanning the Flames (2019)
(Mother Tongue Ink, 2018-19)

Earth Pathways Diary (2013, 2014, 2017, 2018, 2019)

Moon Dreams Diary 2018 (Womancraft Publishing, 2017)

If Women Rose Rooted: a journey to authenticity and belonging,
Sharon Blackie (September Publishing, 2016)

She Rises: how goddess feminism, activism, and spirituality? Volume 2
(Mago Books, 2016)

Wild + Precious: the best of Wild Sister magazine, Jen Saunders
(Wild Sister, 2014)

Tiny Buddha's Guide to Loving Yourself, Lori Deschene (Hay House, 2013)

Roots: where food comes from, and where it takes us (BlogHer, 2013)

Musings on Mothering: an anthology of art, poetry and prose, Teika Bellamy
(Mother's Milk Books, 2012)

*A woman's journey to healing begins the moment she decides
she will no longer abandon herself.*
Amy Bammel Wilding

When women heal, the world heals.
Femme

CONTENTS

ACKNOWLEDGEMENTS

This book was only possible because of those who walked this path before me.

I want to pay heartfelt tribute to my way-showers on this journey: Johanna Hedva, ("Sick Woman Theory"), Charles Eisenstein ("Mutiny of the Soul"), Christiane Northrup (*Women's Bodies, Women's Wisdom*), Kat Duff (*The Alchemy of Illness*), Eve Ensler (*In the Body of the World*) and the many, many others whose work is referenced here. Your powerful writings crystallised for me so many themes that I had been contemplating and living through for most of my adult life. Seeing your courage to confront this topic gave me the permission to finally give voice to my own experience. I am deeply indebted to your valuable, pioneering work. Thank you.

My grandmother Lucy H. Crocker Pearce, a natural philosopher and early female science graduate, whose passion for biology, education and books took bloom first in the Pioneer Health Centre in Peckham, London in the 1930s, and later amongst friends, family and seemingly everyone her life touched. My greatest sadness is that I never got to meet her and never got to see the Peckham Centre. But I carry her name and her spirit. And her passion for health and cultural transformation lives on through all who knew her. I have been lucky enough to be connected directly to it through my parents and my friendship with her co-worker, Elizabeth, a dear friend now in her nineties, who has taught me so much about living well through her own quiet example.

My own dances with healthcare providers have flagged up Western medicine's immense failings and contradictions as well as many deeply compassionate souls who work within its aegises – in hospital emergency departments, inpatient wards, counselling rooms, making appointments, healing with medicine, hands and herbs. I have been blessed by many dear people who have walked beside me in a professional healing capacity and have remained human throughout this journey. Thank you to my real life medicine men and women: Trish, Ines, Jean, Kenny, Conor, Hugh, Seamas and Shirley for consistently going above and beyond, for your intelligence, care and compassion, for showing me what healthcare can and should look like within and beyond the System.

To my women's circles: my women's group that has been my safe space for a decade. And my newer circles: Beth Wallace's women's circles, Cork Asperger's Women's Group and my many Facebook tribes.

To the brave and inspiring women who heard the call on Facebook and gathered as part of the Medicine Woman group, who shared their stories and insight, and who cheered this book on: Kerry Bray, Maddie Millet, Zoë K.M. Foster, Joanne, Lolly Viv Willows, Patrícia Lemos, Ciara Ryan Gerhardt, Joy Horner, Paula Youmell, Michelle Callaghan, Rosie Slosek, Helen, Anna-Maybritt Lamberth, Diana Sette, Bridget Robertson, Lucinda Button, Florence Vion, Tamsin Hopkins, Tess, Charlotte Alling, Ashlee Symington, Aramei Dracharys, Sophie de Carvalho, Sophie Mortimer, Heather Veitch, Anne, Jo Gough, Becky Annison, Marlene Pray, Therese Doherty, Emma Weatherall and Melissa Brown. And to Lewis Barfoot, who gave me massive insight into both sides of the coin.

To my trusted beta-readers: Amy Bammel Wilding, Mary Tighe and Paula Youmell for saying yes. For reading this freshly born book and being brave enough to tell me how to make it better. And to all my generous endorsers.

Tracy Evans, my space holder, idea bouncer, co-conspirator, soul guide, fellow wanderer, resident wise woman and best friend. We did it!

My parents, siblings, husband and kids who have stood by me through thick and thin. Given me space when I needed it, looked after me in my ups and many, many downs, and who have at times been sick and struggling alongside me these past couple of years. We are on this journey together. I am so glad to have your company.

To all the women who, over the years, have read my books, supported my work, believed in me and cheered me on. Who have allowed my words to unfold in their own lives and have trusted me with their stories and secrets in return. To each and every one of you who has made contact to enquire when this book would (finally) be ready: here it is. This is for you.

A PRACTICAL NOTE TO THE READER

Each of my books marks a part of my journey as a cis-white woman, artist and mother living in 21st century patriarchy. I write from my lived and limited perspective for those whom my words resonate with. Each of my books naturally builds on the understanding I have developed in the others, to form a cohesive body of work.

Medicine Woman is envisaged as a companion work to my earlier book, *Burning Woman*. I am aware that I don't want to go over too much of what was already explored in detail in *Burning Woman*, but am also mindful that much of what was said in that book has huge relevance to what is explored here, namely trauma, inflammation, female lineage, epigenetics, birthing practices, our energetic selves and burnout. So, if you have *Burning Woman*, please do reference these sections – they are all, in my mind, interwoven into this puzzle of sickness and transformation. And if you haven't yet read it, then I recommend you do.

Finally, if you are new to my work, or this genre, I point you towards the appendix where I explain my use of certain terms rather than doing so in the main body of the book. Each time a term is raised for the first time you will see an asterisk * alerting you to the fact that you can find out more about it in the appendix. In the appendix you will also find a short section contextualising my own experiences of healthcare and the health system in Ireland, where I live, if you are unfamiliar with it.

①

WHERE WE BEGIN

We begin on the floor of a hospital toilet. A woman lies prostrated, sobbing from her depths. Her child has just been diagnosed with a life-long autoimmune disease. They need to start medication. Today. There are no alternatives. No cures.

The trainee doctor breaks with protocol and strokes the crying child's hair. The mother has been trying to hold it together through meeting after meeting with doctors and nurses in sterile white rooms as they reel off protocols and facts and potential risks in language she barely understands. She slips away to the bathroom and falls to the floor in prayer, distraught: *help us get through this. Make it okay. Please, please, let it be okay.*

That woman is me. That child is mine. Perhaps she is you. Perhaps that child is yours. Perhaps that child was you.

It starts with the little girl whose mother was always sick in bed, and so she learned to be good, to take responsibility for more than her share. She learned to be the one who made things right. She learned to walk on egg shells, to fear what came next, to never trust the good days. She learned not to upset her, not to make her sicker. Believing somehow that her silence would keep her alive. All the while swearing she would never be like her.

Until she too ended up sick in bed.

That child was me. That woman is me. That child is mine. Perhaps that child was you.

It starts in a doctor's consulting room reciting off symptoms, knowing that there are no answers. They cannot help you, they do not know what's wrong, or worse they will mark you down in their own language as delusional: the crazy woman, the worried well, the attention seeker, the hypochondriac, the bored housewife, the hormonal, hysterical or menopausal woman…

That woman is me. Perhaps she is you, your mother, your sister, your daughter, your friend.

This pain is ours.

The suffering is real.

And it has been going on too long.

OPENING

Something is happening under the surface,
Just below the skin.
But we dare not look,
Because we do not know what we might find.
Its presence scares us,
Awakening ghosts we would prefer to disappear.
We stand at the crossroads between old and new, in the place beyond
certainty.
Ready – at last –
To peel back the bandages and look beneath at the raw wounds.
Daring to ask what hurts and why.
And how it might heal.
Without agenda or guarantees or expertise.
With the courage to see
What lies beneath.
Beneath the bulletproof two-way mirror of our cultural narrative,
Into the darkness, the sadness, the pain that we would rather avoid.
In through the blood and the nerves,
To the soul of sickness.

When I was editing my book, *Burning Woman*, in the autumn of 2015, I had whole segments that did not fit. All of them were to do with illness, the sickness of patriarchy* and the need to embody the Feminine* in order to heal ourselves and our world. I put them to one side in a folder marked Medicine Woman and left them. It felt too big, too scary, and I far too small to give voice to what was wanting to come through. My only mistake, although it was really an insurance policy against my own fears winning out, was to announce this book at the end of *Burning Woman*. If I hadn't, or if that book had not turned out to be as successful as it was, I would have backed out of seeing *Medicine Woman* through a hundred thousand times.

As with all my books, I get a title and a knowing of what the book will be, and then I have to live it. This is never my favourite part. I have always found life far easier to manage when it is contained within the covers of other people's books, or figured out analytically, rather than played out in the messy, uncontrolled environs of my own body, mind and daily life.

In *Burning Woman* I birthed my challenge to patriarchal religion and political power. It took every last bit of courage. My adrenaline levels were sky high. I was sick with anxiety, terrified of what the response might be. My life began shrinking as my body and mind could no longer sustain the internal pressure of trying to summon in the new paradigm* whilst inhabiting the old. All the parts of myself that I had tried to suppress, ignore and downplay were coming to the surface once more. I could not run from the truths my body was trying to tell me.

I now know that it was Medicine Woman*, Burning Woman's twin sister, arising within me. But still I tried to run. It's what I've always done, you see, I've never liked confrontation.

But Medicine Woman had my name on her list. My meeting with her was long overdue. In speaking her name aloud, our appointment was set.

I realised that I had been preparing to write this book for most of my adult life. I guess that's why I had forcibly nailed my colours to the mast this time: I had form in backing out.

In my early twenties, after achieving a first class Bachelor's degree in History of Ideas and English Literature, I wrote (but never sent) several university applications for graduate degrees in disciplines spanning the range of healing and medicine from the alternative to the conventional: Jungian Theory; The History of Medicine; Philosophy, Cosmology and Consciousness to name a few. I was wanting something that bridged the worlds of Western* and other medicine. But each time I stepped towards those worlds my fear got bigger: I am not a doctor nor am I wanting to explore these issues in a detached academic manner. I am interested in questioning our current paradigm, understanding the philosophical and historical roots of how we've gotten to where we are... and then helping to shift it to something healthier and more fulfilling. But I did not trust that I would be taken seriously. So, I put the applications aside. And trained to be an English teacher instead.

Medicine Woman did not leave me alone, however. I continued to read avidly on the subject, writing health and healing related articles for a decade on blogs, magazines and national newspapers.

For years I tried to heal theoretically, by reading books, unable to face the pain of the known unknown that waited within. Until the pain was too great and dominated every area of my life. Until it spoke through many of the major biological systems in my body: it was the pain or me that was going to be my everything.

One day, shortly before *Burning Woman* was published, when I was sick in bed once more, two powerful pieces blew my way on the internet within hours of each other – the first, Charles Eisenstein's "Mutiny of the Soul", and the second "The Sick Woman Theory" by Johanna Hedva. I devoured them. Grateful for their daring. For their vision. For their medicine.

I had been sick for years and deeply frustrated with my body. Not hospital sick. But sick enough to have more days ill than well. These two brave spirits reminded me that it was time to embody the healing that I had skirted around for so long. That it was okay to write about it on a more personal and philosophical level. It was okay to question the paradigm we are inhabiting. It was okay to share a vision without having all the answers. In fact, it was more than okay: it was necessary, and urgently so. Not only for myself but all the other incredible people who inhabited the land of the sick: this was much bigger than just me.

In my own life I had begun to get braver in confronting my illness, in trying new healing modalities in a concerted effort to finally figure out what was wrong and get better. I was reading voraciously for my own health and healing and as I traversed the healthcare system I realised that this was a journey I was not walking alone.

Like all of my books, *Medicine Woman* was written as I navigated new terrain in my life, as an offering to myself and all those who might need a companion on a path that is not well-illuminated by our culture.

Each of my books is like a string of prayer beads, threaded with longings, pain, wisdom, poetry and stories of a hundred voices. Each is less a book of answers than a book of questions: a creative weaving of evidence and ideas into the articulation of a dream of how things could be better. It is unapologetically rooted in my own embodied reality and intuitions. My approach has always been to speak from the first-person perspective of the traveller and from the timeless dimensions of the soul, whilst fully grounding my words in a sound foundation of the history of ideas, my undergraduate subject and life-long passion. I call this Living Philosophy.

My books are rooted in the wisdom of many voices, especially female, from across disciplines and cultures. Central to each of my books are the experiences of other women: a living, breathing circle of women who are living the material that I am writing about. You will find their words woven through the book.

When I put out the call online, almost forty women from around the globe gathered to form our original Medicine Woman circle in minutes. I observed in awe as they started to speak: the soul of the book shone through their words. A book they had never read… because it had not yet been published. *Medicine Woman*, the themes and words that I had already noted down, were flowing from their mouths.

I was on the right track. She was real.

I felt humbled and grateful for their openness, for their trust. For many of these women it was the first time sharing so openly about their illness. It was magical to observe how healing spontaneously arose from within themselves when they started to tell their stories, when they began to hear the words of other women and share resources. They felt deep in their bones, perhaps for the first time, that they too were not alone in their suffering. Their conditions may have isolated them from their family of birth, their work, friends, partners or children, but here in the words of other women was belonging. Acceptance. Healing. New ways forward.

It was then that I saw just how dangerous silence is to women's health. And I recognised the true power of words to break the spell of patriarchy and begin the Feminine healing process.

COLLAPSE ON THE WORLD STAGE

As we focused on our personal healing in this private Facebook group, the world around us seemed to be falling apart, its daily monstrosities being shared and anguished over on my Facebook feed.

Whatever your political persuasion, I think you will agree that the intensity and turbulence of the last couple of years has been unprecedented in our lifetimes. Our communities have become deeply fractured and furious from the fall-out from Brexit, #MeToo, the US 2016 election and unprecedented political interference, which have spun Western democracy into far darker, more uncertain places than we have been for a long time. They added fuel and impetus to the fires that were already burning: the massive increase in global terror attacks, the refugee crisis, endemic racism, state brutality, animosity between and within nation states…

Why write a book about sick women, when the world was falling down around our ears, I wondered? What use was it to write a book of hope, when all around services were being cut, when cultural and economic meltdown were in full flow?

But then I realised that the two were intimately connected. I, like so many of us who are empaths or who suffer with mental health issues, found myself struggling against the tide, dealing with the enormity of inhabiting a culture on fire. I noticed how many people on my Facebook feed were having mental and physical health episodes: it was like an explosion of bodies and minds breaking down in synchrony with the last throes of patriarchy. Marriages were collapsing around me. Suicides everywhere I looked. Shootings and more shootings. Instability was rife. Something big was going on in the collective consciousness. Our bodies were freaking out at what our minds were trying hard to block out. Our bodies were not just speaking, they were shrieking. Our systems were collapsing in lockstep with the System*.

Some people would recommend that the cure to this anguish is to get off Facebook and stop watching the news.

But not knowing doesn't stop it happening.

And not everyone is privileged enough to turn off the news: it is their unliveable, lived reality.

COLLAPSE ON THE HOME FRONT

Life wasn't just collapsing online or elsewhere, but on the home front too.

During the writing of this book my family – both within my home, and extended family – experienced more health issues than ever before. Over the space of eighteen months, four out of five of my immediate family received diagnoses of life-long conditions. Several members of our extended families were hospitalised for major health issues. We were left reeling as health disaster after disaster floored many of us in unison, knocking out our support systems, our ability to work, our children's ability to be in school, disrupting our lives beyond recognition and draining our finances and energy…

I entered this journey thinking it was to be my personal journey to take at my own pace. Thinking that healing would hopefully be a story of redemption, love and light. But having successfully avoided and evaded it all my adult life, when I committed to it, it took me down. And hard.

I thought that healing was a reasonably linear path – you find the Truth about what is wrong with you, then you find the Right Path and then you follow it. This may sound simplistic, especially from someone who has spent the best part of twenty years reading about health and healing. But that is what we are sold, by each doctor, each book – follow this protocol, follow it to the letter and you will be cured. We are sold the promise of the cure. The failing when we don't receive it is ours, because we didn't follow the advice to the letter (and to be honest who could?).

I could not have anticipated how complex the healing process would be – how it would impact so many members of our family simultaneously, how it would shake us to our roots so firmly. I got to learn firsthand that the healing process is multidimensional – not only including body, mind and soul* but generations living, dead and unborn, the wider world, the local community and of course the System. It is as complex as solving an invisible Rubik's cube with your hands tied behind your back, which also has temporal dimensions, where each shift impacts all other pieces of the puzzle in unforeseen ways.

Our healing journey over the past two years has encompassed over fifty medical professionals, within both public and private systems, including: family doctors, clinical psychologists, physiotherapists, a psychotherapist, occupational therapists, a dietician, hospital consultants, consultant registrars, many psychiatrists and nurses of many stripes. It has included a veritable alphabet soup of alternative therapies: acupuncture, aromatherapy, art therapy, Body Talk, cannabis oil, cognitive behavioural therapy, cranio-sacral therapy, dietary changes, EFT (tapping), equine therapy, exercise, herbalism, homeopathy, massage, meditation, mindfulness, physiotherapy, psychotherapy, reflexology, rock balancing, sensory processing activities, support groups, women's circles, writing... and many, many different pharmaceutical medications swallowed, injected and spread on the skin. We have received free state healthcare and accessed expensive private care, we have filled in form after form after form for referrals and assessments and state benefits.

Without the writing of this book I am not sure I would have been able to process it all. *Medicine Woman* has been a form of therapy in its own right, to help me, and us, navigate the unknown and find our way towards healing on many levels, beyond that offered by the doctors who have worked so hard on our behalves and yet had so little to offer. We have witnessed the best and worst of what the current medical system has in its bag. And our lives have been crippled by its failings. But nobody died.

Medicine Woman was written on the journey of healing: rooted in the reality of our lives, in the midst of the fear, the uncertainty, the not knowing what will happen, who to trust or what would work. It has been finished many times at many different points in the journey: each time coming to a different conclusion. Writing it has been a way of excavating hope from hopelessness, meaning from meaninglessness and trying to stay connected with the deeper layers of transformation under the daily chaos and overwhelm that so often felt too much to bear.

Sharing our story is a tricky thing. We are real people living in a world where these things are not necessarily talked about. We live in a small community of people I have to see face-to-face, and in a global community of seven billion strangers all connected by the internet. I wanted to be careful to respect my family's privacy, and therefore much of what we have gone through is only alluded to, as theirs are not my stories to tell. In breaking my silence I also break some of theirs. I have tried to do this as unobtrusively as possible whilst also being honest. I hope they, and you, feel I have done this respectfully.

BREAKING SILENCE

One of the core lies of patriarchy is that our suffering is our fault as individuals. It should be borne in silence, so as not to bring others down. When in truth sickness is all around us all the time. It runs down family lines and through communities, it runs along rivers and is carried in the air. Illness – mental or physical – is very rarely an individual thing. It is a deeply human thing, and the shame and fear we carry in silence is an obstacle to our healing.

I need you to know that the fear of speaking up is still big for me. It has stalled this book many times. Again and again the words have dried up. My body has frozen with the fear of breaking the conspiracy of silence that I have been indoctrinated in from all sides in order to be a Good Girl, to stay safe, to wait for permission to speak. A permission that will never come from the System that I need to critique. A permission that can only come from within.

I am aware that what I write may be strange to you. Challenging. Unprovable. Uncomfortable.

The chances are that at some point this book is going to piss you off. Perhaps it already has.

Because what I say or the way I say it will not be exactly what you want to hear. And as a woman I should, our culture tells us, not be offensive or aggressive. I should seek to please you, appease you.

To speak one's subjective truth in one's own raw voice is still subversive. To do it as an unqualified woman doubly so. To speak as a sick woman: don't even bother.

The voice of illness and disability is discomforting to our world, and so it is systematically silenced in deference to the objective, logical, scientific, sterile, patriarchal narrative with which we are more familiar and comfortable. We tend to prefer advocates and charities to speak on behalf of sufferers in cleanly polished corporate-speak. To ensure the safety of our cultural narratives, we deny other ways of healing, speaking and knowing.

From lived experience I have learned that as a heretic and dreamer the requirements of perfection and omniscience are high. I ask your patience and understanding as I pull this vast dream into less than perfect words.

There is often an overwhelming desire in many who are invested in the System to immediately defend it. If you work within Western medicine, or are religious, please know that my argument is with the historical edifices of patriarchy, with unproven prejudice masquerading as Absolute Truth and the Systemic repercussions of this. I am not attacking you as a person. Not your spiritual beliefs. Not your community. Not your heartfelt work for humanity. In these aspects I think you will find us kindred spirits.

For those who have escaped the System (or are trying to), there is often a desire to skip the darkness of the past and jump with both feet into the warm fuzzy hope of healing, so that we can reach the promised land of happily-ever-after. I must warn you now, this book offers no seven-point plan to happily-ever-after. If this is what you are looking for, you may find the first part of this book especially challenging, as it takes us down into the pain that you are trying to avoid by looking at what has gone wrong for us as individuals, as a culture and within Western medicine.

Please beware of skipping ahead because it feels too dark or depressing. Or putting the book down because we do not immediately see eye-to-eye. Trust that you and I and *Medicine Woman* are here for a reason. Something called you here. Hold that above the discomfort you might feel on the journey and dare to dive deep with me.

I believe that we have to see what we have been blind to. We have to hear what we have closed our ears and minds to. We have to start where we are, in order to heal.

That is our shared intention. Let us hold onto that together.

SPEAKING FOR THE FEMININE

Why focus exclusively on women? What about all the men? I am regularly asked. *They are sick too*, I am told. As though I don't have a beloved husband, father or son who are sick too. As though I don't have three brothers. And countless male friends, each fighting their own health battles in this world. *Don't you care about them?*

I care deeply. And much of what I write is applicable to all genders. Much of the healing we need is because we are human, inhabiting a broken, inhumane System.

But I want to dedicate my energy to breaking the silence and invisibility that has been used to deny the reality of women's lives and experiences, historically and systematically. I want to make space for women's perspectives. Women's experiences. Women's bodies. Women's voices. Women's suffering. Women's stories. Women's sickness. I want to give voice to a vision of a world that honours us all. I want to make sacred space for the experience of being a woman in this world, and especially for the sick women in a sick world.

It is to this lack that I write.

Bodies have always been problematic: culturally, philosophically and biologically in their reluctance to be constrained by the simplicity of words. Women's bodies even more so. I know that there are many who wish to move beyond the binary terms of man and woman, masculine and feminine, and into the fullness of gender fluidity in infinite forms. I am open to the freedoms and possibilities that this new paradigm may hold. I embrace the rights and needs of each individual to be respected as it emerges. And yet, there remains the fact that the paradigm we inhabit is still, and has historically been, gendered. Bodies have belonged, and still do, in the clear majority, to two sexes.

My heart is in it for all of us to find health. We cannot heal one sex and not the other. But our histories have been so different, our bodies are different, our gendered roles are still different. And I'm sick and tired of women being told that we're equal, so stop whining, when it suits society, yet in underhanded, subtle ways being told we are weak, crazy, hysterical hypochondriacs in a world that doesn't understand our bodies and tends to be less able to treat them when they are sick.

What I and countless other women have found as we have struggled with our health is that there are often few who can see us, few who will speak for us, few who really understand what is going on in our bodies and minds. And when they do there is little they can do for us. Because our sickness *is* a gendered problem.

Many times in this book you will find ways that I have generalised the experience of 'woman' or 'man' that do not apply to every person of that gender that you know. That may not relate to you. In the act of writing and being able to speak some truths that I have not heard spoken before, generalisations will be made. Please know I do not claim to speak for *you*. I cannot speak *your* truth. Only you can. And I encourage you to do so. I am one woman, with one perspective. It is my intention that in speaking my truth I hold space for you to speak yours, so that this new cultural narrative is woven from many, many voices that have previously been marginalised. In breaking my silence my dearest wish is that I make it a little easier for you to break yours.

You will notice that I share the voice of the Feminine in many ways: through personal journal-like entries and poetry, as well as the voices of other women, alongside the more familiar non-fiction elements of prose and footnoted factual research. Some of these forms of expression may make you uncomfortable – I know they can still make me feel that way. You may also experience a felt sense of jarring as you shift gears between one part of your knowing and another that these forms engender. Please know this is intentional. I believe all ways of knowing – intuitive and free-flowing, linear and logical – are needed. This is the underlying premise of this book, of all my work. But we are not used to this. And so it can seem strange.

To give voice to the Feminine – those values and qualities which our culture has attributed to females, considered of less importance to dominant masculine values – and to speak for the female body and soul is usually pretty unpopular and unfashionable for a whole host of different reasons. It is to centre the subjugated, speak the unspeakable and to break with orthodoxy. It is to question the accepted narrative of the dominant System in an unfamiliar language. It is to try to name the invisible miasma within which we exist. To do so is to risk being branded crazy, ridiculous, irresponsible, irrelevant or hysterical.

It is a risk I am prepared to take.

I know it would be easier for those invested in the System if this book could be dismissed as the ramblings of a crazy lady, rather than a harbinger of truth.

I leave it to you to decide.

TO HEALING

Medicine Woman speaks to healing on many levels. It is a narrative of my own healing journey and a handbook to emotionally and practically support the healing of others. It does this not just through providing insight or information, but through using words as medicine: narrative itself as a medium for healing and creativity as a mode for transforming pain.

If *Burning Woman* was a declaration of the power of a woman's spirit, *Medicine Woman* is a woman's declaration of independence over her own bodymind*: an outrageous reclaiming of our power to heal ourselves.

I thought this was a book about why we were getting sick, but rather it is a book about redefining and reclaiming our lives and our health. It is a call to power for women to stand up for ourselves within the System and to help co-create a healthier system. It is not intended as a wholesale rejection or refusal of Western medicine. Rather it is a refusal of the continued supremacy of the hallowed, unquestionable institution of patriarchal medicine that is philosophically, financially, energetically and ecologically unsustainable in its current form.

My speaking out has already caused ripples of healing within my communities. And with the publication of this book, I hope these ripples will spread further. That through these words, the dream of something big and brave and new may reach us all. That it may inspire and bolster our work for a culture in which healing is more humane and holy. For me, for you, for our children, for the generations to come, and for the world which is our home.

SYMPTOMS: WHAT'S WRONG?

WHAT'S WRONG WITH ME?

Somewhere I lost myself.
I lost the beat of my heart as my own drum.
I have a sense that it was the same time I lost Medicine Woman.
One day my soul slipped out of my body.
Or maybe it was pulled too hard. Or shocked away.
I don't know.
All I know is that I lost her,
And have been sick ever since.
An orphaned child
In a world that does not feel like home.
I have been wandering
Lost…
Wondering…
Where do you go when your body is broken?
Who can you call on when your mind is shattered into a thousand pieces,
When your skin is on fire and your soul is nowhere to be found?

These thoughts spin around my head in the quiet of night when I lie awake too frazzled to sleep.

What's wrong with me? Who can help me?

I try to take each day at a time, but my mind races forwards. I am sick of being sick, but I can see no way out. The sting of not being believed, of being thought to be a hypochondriac, is worse than if something's seriously wrong.

I am not as sick as many. I should be grateful for all I have. I start to list my blessings: a warm home, a loving partner, three children, a good education, work I am passionate about, food in the fridge, all my fingers and toes, a car, enough money in the bank for the next few weeks, a safe community in a safe country...

Focus on the positives. Be grateful.

I am. I know none of these things are to be taken for granted. I am immensely privileged. This is part of the reason I give myself such a hard time. I think of all those around the world suffering in much worse ways than me. People dying of cancer, in wars, of AIDS, of malaria and typhoid, people being beaten and tortured and starving...

But their greater suffering does not eliminate mine. I am not imagining it. Something is most definitely not right within me.

What's wrong with me?

I try to keep it to myself. Sometimes (often) I type my symptoms into Google. I ask friends. Read books. Try herbs. Exercise. Vitamins. Meditate. Read some more.

Mostly I just try to put the pain and exhaustion to the back of my mind. Pop a painkiller and carry on as usual: school runs, grocery shopping, panic attacks, play-dates, work, migraine, laundry, hospital trips, art...

Then after months and months of going through it in my head, when I'm feeling particularly brave or disturbed or bewildered or broken, I find myself sitting in a chair in a small white room, with a pot plant on the desk beside the computer, asking my doctor.

What's wrong with me?

I have huge liking for my doctor, he's a champion of breastfeeding and homebirth in a conservative system that is suspicious of both. He's a kind man with a big heart who knows what it's like to be dealt a hard hand. But in the rushed moments we have together he can barely get the smallest grasp on the complex tapestry that is my health. We both know there is little that he has within his power to treat or cure me. But still I come to him for answers to the question that plays on repeat in my mind.

What's wrong with me?

I long for a simple solution. For a magic bullet. A cure. A label so that I know what I'm dealing with and can explain to others what my life is like on the inside. A magic wand would be nice. Something, anything, to make me better. But he has none. Just a caring manner, another battery of blood tests that come out okay-ish – a little low on this and a little high on that, but nothing to get excited about. Nothing conclusive. Nothing serious. Nothing. Apparently.

What's wrong with me?

He is scratching the surface, missing all the knotted complexities of trauma and genetics and my childhood medical history in another country. Unable to see the various layers of the sickness in his tests. He writes a prescription. Even though we both know I probably won't take it. He is trying his best to help, not knowing what he's really treating. Knowing that his medicines work for some and not others. And usually not for me.

His medicines usually make me sicker. Really sick. Scary sick. And so I am caught in limbo. There's nothing he can treat with what he has available to him. He holds no cures for me, but my bodymind insists something is wrong.

What's wrong with me?

And so I turn elsewhere, encouraged by friends and acquaintances who have lost faith in the System. We don't have enough money to try a full immersion in alternative therapies, I do not trust anything too woo-woo anyway. I need my alternatives to be grounded in evidence not wishful thinking. I cannot afford to take time from work for constant appointments. And so I dip my toe in here and there.

Some recommend visualisations and affirmations as they work on my aching muscles and joints and prescribe their own tinctures and tablets.

I can heal myself.

I pronounce, as I stand in the firelight, believing, hoping, for that moment, that the New Age folks are right. Maybe my sickness is all in my mind. Maybe I can just think myself better.

I can heal myself.

My illness had just been bad thinking. Weakness. Victim mentality. Low vibrations. Just a story I had been telling myself. I could consciously let go of it and be free. All I had to do was choose to be healthy. Think positive. Focus on the good. On love and light.

I am healed.

I declare. Waiting for the thunderbolt. Trying desperately to imagine golden light coming down from above, my roots deep in the soil…

I am vibrant. I am healthy. I am strong.

My back is aching. Legs are shaking. Heart racing.

I am vibrant. I am healthy. I am strong.

Where the medical profession cannot find anything wrong, practitioners in alternative health fields say that everything is…

The problem is… your gut microbiome. Negative thinking. Hormone imbalance. Lumbar subluxations. Chi blockage in your liver. Energetic frequencies in your home. Parasites. Mineral deficiencies. Candida overgrowth. Your subconscious.

All these assertions are possible… but not provable. So I have to choose whether to put my trust and my money in their hands or not.

It all feels like stabbing in the dark. And I just want to know what this is for sure … and get better, at last.

What is wrong with me?

Perhaps sickness was just my way of hiding from the world. Of getting pity from others. Or wanting to be special. People had said variations of these things to me over the years.

Just like they had to my mother before me. I could get better just as soon as I made the choice to. The power to heal was my own decision.

I am vibrant. I am healthy. I am strong.

For most of my childhood there was always something wrong with her. The minor things took her attention, the major things seemed to slip under the doctors' radars. She never had any real answers. Just constant questions that her body inhabited as illness.

I have the power to change.

I grew up swearing I would not be like her, whilst constantly being sick. My father couldn't bear me being sick. Something about this weak state made him deeply uncomfortable. Death and he were always uncomfortable bed-fellows. He wanted me to be active and outgoing, confident and positive: brave, strong and fearless like him. He regularly pointed out to me that I was *just like my mother* when I was sick.

This was never a good thing.

They got sick of each other early on. My world split in two at the beginning of my life. Two lands, two homes, two worlds. I was always scared on a level beyond words that they would get sick of me. That my problems would become A Problem. So I hid them as much as possible. Learned to keep things to myself (though they always spilled out in unbidden tears). Tried to be strong. To carry on. To push myself.

Don't be needy.

I am strong and healthy.

I hid from my sickness. From this weak feminine self. I denied it as best I could. Until my sick self got bigger and bigger and I could no longer hide it under the bed. I could not function any more and took to my bed during the day.

It's all in my mind… it's all in my mind…

I have many of the same issues my mother had. And that made me really mad. Because either I was recreating her existence subconsciously: I had learned how to be sick, it was all in my mind, just like it was with her. Or maybe, and this was worse, there was a lot wrong with me, and had been with her, and medical science didn't get it. Couldn't see it. We were invisible to them. Our suffering illusory.

I create my own reality.

And then my daughter started presenting with certain struggles, which the doctors and teachers didn't recognise, but I did. They thought we were imagining it. Told us so. Again and again. Three generations. Maybe more. Disbelieved. Suffering.

There's nothing wrong. Nothing. Wrong. Nothingwrongnothingwrongnothingwrong.

It's all in your mind.

Focus on the positive.

What I struggle with is multifarious and shifting: depression, anxiety, sky-high stress levels, panic attacks, migraines, long-term lower back and pelvic problems, exhaustion, itching skin, regular swollen glands, severe brain fog, almost constant low-grade infections, chronic digestive issues, joints that shift painfully out of place on a regular basis when yawning or sneezing or getting out of bed or having sex or walking on uneven ground, high cholesterol, cold body… and did I mention exhaustion? And anxiety?

What's wrong with me?

Life overwhelms me on a daily basis. Normal is what I have always pushed myself to be, to achieve, but have fallen far short of. I can't do normal life the way most people seem to be able to. And these last few years have not been normal by anybody's parameters. The levels of stress that we have been living under on a daily basis in our family home have been unbearable. But still I have tried to carry on. Taking the blame for being sick. Taking the blame for my kids being sick. Trying to hold it all together. To keep the show on the road. Working harder and harder and harder to sustain an appearance of normality.

There's nothing wrong. Don't make a fuss.

I find being sick all the time deeply frustrating. Where my mum had spent most of her life devoted to us kids and the home, sick and overwhelmed, I wanted more. I wanted to be an artist, a creative entrepreneur like my father and uncle, not just confined by motherhood. I built a career as a writer. We built two businesses. To the outside world it looked like I had it sorted. I was driven. Getting successful.

It's just I was always in bed. Sick.

There's nothing wrong. Don't make a fuss.

But I wasn't going to let sickness stop me. So I worked from bed. Refusing to give in to the weakness of my body. Angry and frustrated at myself. Caged in by anxiety and exhaustion. Running on fear and adrenaline. Trying to outrun my sickness. Not knowing how to get better. Not knowing what was wrong or who could help me.

I was sick of being sick and wanted to be able to dive into my life.

What's wrong with me?

It wasn't a new thing. I have been sick all my life, with regular long-distance trips to expensive ear, nose and throat specialists as a young child. Constant antibiotics. When they failed a dairy-free diet and nasty tasting herbal remedies were my normal. Homeopaths and osteopaths a common day out for me. I was always sicker than others. Not dying sick, I've never had an operation, just not well. But certainly not imagining things. Colds and flu and tonsillitis and gastrointestinal bugs are not figments of the imagination – they go around families and social groups. And I always seem to get every one. And get it hardest. Prozac was recommended at sixteen. The Pill was prescribed for acne and fainting and hormonal issues too. Later beta blockers. Antidepressants. Anti-anxiety medications. Lots of antibiotics. Pills but no answers.

What's wrong now?

I am thirty-seven. Sickness peaks again. I am bone tired. I have nowhere to turn. I am so angry. At myself. At everyone. And so I do the only thing I have never done. The thing I have never been able to afford to do: stop. Drop everything. (Well, as much as I can as a self-employed mother of three with no childcare can.) And really listen to my bodymind. Dare to look into the dark places I have been avoiding. Dedicate myself to compassionately unravelling the mystery of my body's full story, with love and patience and care. Giving myself the time and space I need to heal. Building the team of healing allies I need to help me find the answers that have lain hidden.

In the midst of feeling ill, I feel desperately alone. But on the days I feel a little weller, I notice I am not. Why are so many women – women supposedly in the prime of life – sick? And tired. All the time.

What's wrong with us?

There is a massive community of sick women: playing body detective, reflecting on the meaning of what is happening, looking for hope, for healing, for allies, for a broader definition of wellness. Having to abandon our old lives and finally listen to our bodies insistence that...

Something's wrong.

In our bodies, in the world.

For years we have felt powerless. Ashamed. Alone. Unsure of how to proceed, who to trust. Scared that we will be shamed for our sickness, for our inability to get better.

Something's wrong.

It seems we have imbibed the story of Cassandra subconsciously. You may never have heard her legend before in your classroom or at your grandmother's knee, I certainly hadn't. But we know it in our bones.

Cassandra was a woman who was gifted by the god Apollo with the ability to prophesy. She spoke aloud what was going to happen. But no one believed her prophecies: they were too disturbing to the comfortable reality of those around her. And so she was confined to the care of a warden, driven mad from being disbelieved. Again and again she warned them...

Something's wrong. Something's very wrong.

But they did not listen. They could not hear.

The painful irony was that it was not really the *truth* that people could not heed. It was that it came through the body and voice of a *woman. That* was unbearable.

You see, Cassandra instructed her twin brother in the power of prophecy. Unlike his sister, people believed him. People listened to him when he said:

Something's wrong. Something's very wrong.

We are the Cassandras of our world, gifted with highly sensitive bodies that are feeling what the System would have us ignore. We have been taught to distrust our own body systems, to distrust our inner knowing, to hand over their care and definition to the experts.

We have grown up seeing the women around us consistently disempowered, sick in body or soul, heart or mind. Hearing their suffering dismissed, in big ways and small. Witnessing their physical and emotional needs go unrecognised and unmet for generations. We have grown up feeling alienated from our own bodies, embarrassed or ashamed of them, not at home in our physical selves. We have learned to turn down our emotional responses. We have silenced ourselves, blamed ourselves, punished ourselves.

We have internalised the message that there's something wrong with *us*, rather than there is something *wrong*.

Listen carefully.

Something is wrong. Something's very wrong.

It is time for us to change the story.
And it starts with us.

I'M FINE

You ask me how I am, and I say: *fine.*

Under *fine* lies this…

I just managed to do a solo work trip away – my first event in two years because of anxiety.

Can I do it?

The month before the trip I was ill in bed more days than not. I didn't think I'd be able to do it, but the tickets were booked and people were expecting me.

I have to do it.

On the first two days of the trip I work through *Medicine Woman* with my structural editor and have a massive panic attack as we dig into the trauma that lies below it. I drive a couple of hours through a city I have never driven before and set up my book stall at the conference.

I can do it.

The next day I do the stall and my first public talk in years. I set off home the day after. On the ferry I sit elated. Proud of myself.

I did it, I did it!

And then my neck starts to tense, head to ache – a migraine is hitting in. The ferry crossing is rough, people around me are vomiting. I take painkillers and feel really nauseous but put it down to the migraine and the storm. I lie down and try to sleep. Just before arrival I vomit again and again. The last call for drivers to go back to their cars is sounding. My legs are shaking and I'm sobbing. I get into the car to start the last leg of this mammoth eleven-hour journey. There's just two and a half hours to go, it's getting dark, I just want to be home. To collapse.

I can do it…

Waves of nausea hit me as I drive, the car lights disorienting me. I open the window, breathe deep, focus on the countdown of the satnav timer. I don't want to be a sick woman by myself in the dark on the side of the motorway.

I can do it…

I make it home and say hello as I run past into the bathroom and vomit until my stomach is empty again. Feeling guilty that my body is so weak. That I'm being a bad mother after several days away. All I want is to go to bed.

I'm done.

I vomit through the night and delegate work for the day. My lower back and hip ache is building to a crescendo, my hypermobile joints flaring because of premenstrual hormone levels. My stomach cramps and aches each time I try to eat or drink. I hear tension brewing downstairs and so begins an hour of calming a meltdown. And then another the next morning. I am exhausted and shaking.

I can't do it.

I have to do it.

Today is the online launch of our new book. I do it from the comfort of bed with the electric blanket up high to soothe my aching joints, grateful once again that I am self-employed. Wishing once again that I could have a paid sick day. I flick between internet browser windows, anxiously checking the news to see if World War Three has erupted. I manage to secure an emergency physio appointment, she puts me back into place but bruises me massively in the process.

I get my period, feeling dull and sad and heavy. The whole of my lower body aches. I spend the rest of the day in bed working, with a hot water bottle on my belly to ease the pains, getting up when the kids are home from school to do homework and dinner.

I'm done.

The next morning I wake super-early from anxiety dreams, have a panic attack as silently as I can in the bathroom without waking the house. Another morning, another meltdown. School uniforms, packed lunches…

I try to go for a gentle walk on the beach with my husband but my body is too sore, and I have to turn around after five minutes.

I can't do it.

Day three of my period. I wake with a splitting headache, do breakfasts and school lunches, go back to bed when the painkillers don't work. I attempt a little work and prepare for our mother-daughter circle this evening. On the way home one daughter twists her ankle badly. Ice, painkillers, kids to bed, tooth under pillow. I wake in the middle of the night with a migraine. Again. I take painkillers. Again.

I'm done. Properly, completely, absolutely done.

But I'm not. I've been asleep for an hour when our diabetic child wakes vomiting. I sit up with them till 4am – clearing vomit, piling up soiled sheets, disinfecting surfaces, reassuring, soothing, checking blood sugar levels. I wake in the morning with the migraine still blaring. Re-check daughter's ankle for breakage. Just a sprain. More ice. More painkillers. Phone the hospital needing support in managing child's Type 1 diabetes with vomiting bug and am required to phone back hourly to check in with the nurse. I continue checking ketones and blood sugars, administering fluids, trying to stave off hospitalisation. It doesn't work.

Help!

We head to the emergency room. Drip for fluids. Home again. Dinner. Everyone decompressing after the stress. Meltdowns. Tears. Hugs. Bed.

I'm so far beyond done I no longer know who I am.

The tooth fairy didn't come again and Santa is borderline suicidal.
You ask how my week was.
This is how it was.
And this is not unusual.
This is my life.
So you ask me how I am, and I smile weakly, and I say,
Fine
Because you do not want to hear this tale of woe, because there's nothing you can do to make it better, because it sounds too much. *It is too much.*

Because depending on your relationship with me, telling you will make me into a moaner, a victim. Or it will make me unreliable. Unprofessional.

I cannot tell you the details, because sickness should be borne privately, unless it is life-threatening, and still then, it should be white-washed, kept secret.

I cannot tell you because you want to hear the victory tale of the famous author who just went on an exciting work trip. Not the human woman who is sick and crumbling.

I cannot tell you because I don't want to burst into tears and make a scene in public.

There's nothing that you can do to make it better. Nothing I can do. We each have our own struggles, our own cross to bear.

And so you ask me how I am.

And I avert my eyes and say *fine*. And try to smile.

Sometimes it works. And sometimes when I try it in the psychiatrist's chair, and she tries to push past *fine*, it doesn't. I am unable to find the words, the tears stream down my face, I start to rock and hyperventilate.

She asks if someone died.

No one died.

Everything's fine really. Except it's not.

I am so done with this. With everything. I cannot carry on, cannot live like this anymore.

I have lived my whole life behind the mask of *fine*. Most of us have. It is what is expected of us, needed of us.

Fine, nothing to see here.

Fine, let's get off this uncomfortable subject.

Fine, let's carry on as normal.

We don't know how to deal with the mess, the discomfort, the hurt, the trauma behind the carefully crafted persona.

Until one day the mask is ripped away. And *fine* is no longer possible.

Sickness finally forces us to drop the performance of superficial strength. It requires us to stop being who we were pretending to be, who we wanted to be.

It insists that we, at last, be who we are.

Once the mask has gone, healing can begin.

WHAT'S WRONG WITH US?

The world around me is failing,
But they can't see.
They say that everything's normal,
And there's something wrong with me.

If we want to heal, and heal deeply, we need to take some time to explore honestly what is going on underneath our superficial performance of normality – individual and collective – to see how things *really* are and how we got here.

This is not an approach we are comfortable with or used to in our quick-fix society, which is captivated with papering over the cracks, rather than examining root causes.

When we turn up at our overflowing doctors' surgeries and emergency rooms we are treated as individuals: considered anomalies of ill health within a healthy context.

We are not.

That is our first, and rather crucial, mistake.

And it's one I know well, from personal experience. You see, when I started out, I thought this book was about what was *wrong* with *me*, why I was failing at wellness. I was angry and confused: I am intelligent, well-educated and well-resourced, I try to live well and take care of myself, but still I am sick much of the time.

But I realised I was far from alone in this. The women that I know in real life and social media, who are some of the long-term sick of the world, are also some of the most clever, creative, inspiring, compassionate, loving, hard-working, visionary people I know.

They are sick, but they are not the losers that our culture insists that sick people are. They are not stupid or uneducated. They are not living extreme lifestyles or bringing their sickness on themselves. No, they are relatively privileged and wealthy in historical and global terms. They are not slackers, spongers, attention-seeking fantasists or hysterical.

They are bold and brave and strong and caring. And totally exhausted. They are good people who do good things in this world… but who find it hard to live in it because of its damaging effect on their systems.

There are a lot of us in this boat.

Sick and not getting better. Unable to live the way we are. Despairing. Alone. Undiagnosed or undiagnosable by our doctors. Untreated or untreatable by Western medicine.

And this is deeply frustrating. Because Western medicine has been an incredible boon for humanity in general in so many ways: treating previously untreatable conditions very effectively from many cancers, to broken bones, to reconstructive surgery and transplants. Anaesthesia, analgesics and antibiotics have lengthened our lifespans and reduced suffering. In terms of life-saving and acute medical treatment I would rather live today than at any other era in human history. I am deeply grateful for it.

But beneath the radar of massive advances in medical science and technology, there is a silent global epidemic, one that is rarely reported with panic: the fast-growing number of chronically ill women of the Western world.

Despite an ever-increasing arsenal of medications and operative techniques, despite our collective wealth and extended lifetimes, chronic illness has become the new norm. Particularly amongst women aged thirty to fifty.

In many cases these illnesses are not immediately life-threatening, but they are life-changing: draining the energy, resources and abilities of the sufferers and profoundly impacting their daily lives. These women who are – or 'should' be – working, creating, childbearing, child-caring, elder-caring, community building, thriving are instead exhausted, bed-ridden, house-bound and debilitated.

But there is no outcry.

Instead as our numbers increase, the doctors' understanding of the causes of these illnesses and how to treat them remains static and the cures seem stalled.

A NEW LIFE

Night becomes wakeful, daytime a blur. Unencumbered by the milestones of work and meals to tether it, time runs like a river, whilst standing firm like a mountain.

Sick time is not clock time, but an alternate binary reality of

Pain/no pain.

Pain/no pain.

Pain/no pain.

You take on a new nationality: patient.

Impatient, you long

For your citizenship of this strange land to be revoked

To return home

To food that tastes right and words you can follow.

Instead your new terrain takes you from one side of your bed to the other. Outer seasons and weather are replaced by the ravages of inner storms and the landscape of pain. Your energy no longer gushes like a newly bored oil-well but is measured in spoons.

Some of us fall through the unseen cracks in the world of health on a bright summer's day through a run-in with machine or microbe, like Alice down the rabbit hole. Some of us were born this way. And some discover that our genes have hidden within them a ticking time bomb. Waiting. Silently.

However we got here, we find ourselves unwillingly inhabitants of the state of sickness. Our papers for the world of health have been rescinded without notice. Though we all know logically that the land of the dead will be our final resting place, its halfway house, the state of sickness, always seems a surprise. We were not taught its customs, its ways.

We never thought we would have to make this our home.

THE RISE AND RISE OF AUTOIMMUNE CONDITIONS

The evidence is fast becoming clear: chronic disease affects women and men differently. But this is relatively new knowledge: until recently, most research on chronic disease did not take sex and gender into account.[1]

Canadian Women's Health Network

We are, it seems, literally and metaphorically becoming allergic to the world we have created... and to our own bodies.

Of the 50 million Americans (that is nearly 20% of the population) with an autoimmune disease, more than 75% of them are women.[2] Autoimmune conditions – which occur when the body recognises one of its own organs as a foreign body and mobilises an immune response against it – are the fourth largest cause of disability in American women.[3]

There are well over a hundred autoimmune conditions. Most of them discovered in the past century. And rates are growing exponentially. Cases of Type 1 diabetes have doubled in the past twenty years.[4] The number of patients with lupus has tripled in the United States over the same period, and women are nine times more likely than men to suffer from it.[5] Multiple sclerosis rates have doubled in that time in many European countries, and it is twice as common in women as men. Fibromyalgia is rocketing: according to the American College of Rheumatology, 3-5% of women in the US now have it, with female rates being seven times higher than in men.[6] Hashimoto's, an autoimmune condition of the thyroid, is 90% more common in women. Graves', another thyroid condition, is seven times more prevalent in women.[7] Coeliac disease is over three times more common, and usually more severe, in women and the age of diagnosis is lower.[8]

This growth in autoimmune conditions is unprecedented. And they are striking down more and more women each year. So where's the public health awareness? Where are the government debates as to what's happening? Where is the money being pumped into research? Where are the treatments? Where are the support services?

Good questions! Instead of an outcry there is doubt and denial, from the medical profession and from the general population.

As Meghan O'Rourke points out, this has been part of their history: "From the start, the study of autoimmunity has been characterized by uncertainty and error. In 1901, the influential German immunologist Paul Ehrlich argued that autoimmunity couldn't exist, because the body had a fear of self-poisoning. Ehrlich's theory was so fully embraced that doctors stopped exploring the subject for half a century."[9]

And it seems that little has changed, as the American Autoimmune Related Diseases Association (AARDA) notes, "Despite the statistics, autoimmune diseases remain among the most poorly understood and poorly recognized of any category of illness."[10]

Whilst some autoimmune conditions have only been identified in the past century, others, like Type 1 diabetes, have been around for much of human history. No one denies the reality of diabetes. No character flaw or assertion of psychosomatics is assigned to its emergence in a body. It is relatively simple to test for and diagnose, and treatment protocol is well-established, although it is an arduous life-long condition to manage. I know this all too well, as one of our children was diagnosed with it during the process of writing this book. But Type 1 diabetes, as well as being known about for longer, also has a simpler biological effect, and, perhaps most importantly... "both sexes are equally affected in childhood, but men are more commonly affected in early adult life."[11] The money, it seems, goes where the men are.

But for many other (predominantly female) autoimmune conditions there is no systematic tool for diagnosis, no definitive blood test and no straightforward treatment protocol. And this lack of medical ability to diagnose along with the fact that most of the symptoms are invisible to the outside observer, tends to lead to disbelief of the patient's suffering. Predominantly women's suffering.

According to a recent AARDA survey, "over 45% of patients with autoimmune diseases have been labelled chronic complainers in the earliest stages of their illness."[12] In the tragic words of one autoimmune sufferer, Meghan O'Rourke: "One way to tell the story is to say that I was ill for a long time – at least half a dozen years – before any doctor I saw believed I had a disease."[13]

Many times women only get diagnosis after years of exhaustive personal research and self-advocacy. Go and see your family doctor and it is unlikely that you will find out what's wrong straight away.

According to Maya Dusenbery in her book, *Doing Harm*, it takes "an average of twelve months for men to get diagnosed with Crohn's disease, an autoimmune disease of the gastrointestinal tract, compared to twenty months for women. Men were diagnosed with Ehlers-Danlos syndrome, a group of genetic disorders that affect the connective tissue, in four years. For women: sixteen years."[14]

It takes, on average, 4.6 years to be diagnosed with an autoimmune condition.[15] Almost five years. Of persistence, self-doubt, desperation and suffering, of endlessly advocating for yourself and questioning the authorities. Years of expensive appointments or long waiting lists for referrals. And five doctors. For many women, especially on lower incomes and women of colour, it may be twice as long as this. Or even longer. And at the end you may well receive a diagnosis which many health professionals and relatives will still scorn. And little help in the way of effective treatment.

This has been the case for so many complex 'invisible' conditions suffered by (predominantly) women over the years: ME, fibromyalgia, chronic fatigue, rheumatoid arthritis as well as other conditions such as Lyme disease, migraine, Ehlers-Danlos syndrome and many neurological conditions including bipolar, Asperger Syndrome, depression, anxiety and post-traumatic stress disorder. And what about the mushrooming of other chronic conditions: asthma and eczema, as well as allergies from hay fever to dust mites, to gluten and lactose intolerance? Until these were finally, formally 'discovered' by the men in white coats over the course of the twentieth century, these sufferings were ignored, trivialised and dismissed, written down to nerves, hysteria, hypochondria, attention seeking... Still today their treatment is patchy at best. Especially for women.

....

The whole of the history of medicine is stuffed with the results of men treating women as second-class persons. If men were treated as badly by male doctors, there'd be an outcry you'd be able to hear on the moon.
ANNETTE

....

It is not just that these illnesses are hard to diagnose. There is also huge controversy between experts within the medical profession, and even more so between the warring factions of the medical and alternative fields of healing, as to what is even real, let alone how to treat them.

Our doctors, it seems, were not trained for what they are being presented with. Their training has prepared them for discrete, known diseases that have been around for centuries, caused by definable pathogens or accidents: cancer, heart disease, kidney stones, gout, broken bones or strokes. Not these conditions that affect multiple systems, wilfully traversing the body and mind, flaring up at irregular and unpredictable intervals over the course of a lifetime, invisibly depleting energy levels and mental focus.

Once you get outside of the realm of having just one discrete condition, good luck to you. If you have multiple co-morbidities that complicate the picture, if your suffering and symptoms do not fit any exact model, then you're on your own.

In too many cases the hard-to-diagnose patient is blacklisted for being too complex, too demanding or not getting better. The general consensus is not "shit, what is happening?" but "it's shit, it's not happening." And so doctors and layfolk alike tend to treat the rising numbers of women with previously rare conditions as a sign that women are attention-seeking, or that doctors have lowered the diagnostic thresholds. Certainly what is happening is not *just* an increase in sickness. Some of the rise of diagnoses in autoimmunity and autism can be attributed to a combination of better diagnostic tools and better-informed patients. But not all.

Something is happening, the numbers of those with chronic conditions are growing exponentially, and the honest answer is, the scientists do not know why.

Western medicine, it seems, has little to say about the illnesses that cross boundaries – that are one part allergy, two parts long-term trauma, three parts environmental aggravation, four parts autoimmune, five parts stress, with a large dash of gender issues, genetics, soul sickness, energy depletion and cultural malaise thrown in for good measure.

One of the reasons that professionals are not 'getting it' is perhaps that they are only seeing a part of the process, rather than the end result. As women move from doctor to doctor looking for diagnoses, the earlier doctors may not hear of the final findings, as Maya Dusenbery found during her research: "I was surprised to realize just how little feedback doctors receive on their diagnostic errors. There hasn't been much systematic research looking into misdiagnoses and delayed diagnoses. A woman with an autoimmune disease may go to four different doctors, and the doctors who didn't properly diagnose her may just see her as a stressed woman and don't get the memo down the road when she's properly diagnosed. It becomes a self-perpetuating problem that feeds into the stereotype that women are just stressed-out hypochondriacs."[16] The same is most certainly true of autistic women.

But if you do your own research online, trying to put together the pieces yourself, you will be told, most likely, when you come back to your doctor with your self-diagnosis, that adrenal fatigue or autistic burnout are not real things. Even though millions of women believe that they are suffering from them, thanks to symptom checklists and treatment protocols found on the internet. Multiple chemical sensitivities are deemed questionable. Candida overgrowth is a fantasy of hippie herbalists. Epstein-Barr syndrome is made up by quacks. Ditto chronic fatigue.

And so we find ourselves in the situation where hundreds of millions of women around the world are falling through the Western medical net. Unaware of what might be wrong with them. Too sick to function normally, not sick enough to get what treatment there is. Unable to get diagnosis, or not able to access it because of service cuts, a lack of professionals in their area or funds to access therapies.

What does it mean when hundreds of millions of women around the world cannot live normal lives because of untreated long-term health conditions? If you add together the number of women with mental health issues to the number with autoimmune diseases in America (38 million) – that's what you get. Add on the 28 million women who suffer from migraine. Adjust for the multiple women who suffer from autoimmune, mental health and migraine and you're at around 50 million women. Just in America. And the same is being echoed in countries across the world.

As the Western way of living spreads, so too do our illnesses. There is a sickness at the heart of our culture, and we've exported it around the world. But we can't, or won't, diagnose what it is.

WHAT'S MAKING US SICK?

*Some days I just don't have the energy to hide that
I am devastated by this illness.*
The Unchargeables

So what is causing this incredible rise in illness? The short answer is: nobody knows for sure. The possible explanations are many.

The state of our environment is most definitely a factor, that much is admitted by governments and health agencies. Especially recently with regard to air pollution levels and respiratory illness. According to a 2018 report from the UK Office for National Statistics, deaths from asthma in London have risen 25% in a decade, and by 43% in the 55-64 age group in the previous two years.[17]

Also implicated are the ever-greater numbers of chemicals, hormones and hormone-mimicking chemicals that have infiltrated every aspect of our environment from the food we eat, to the air we breathe, the water we drink and the land we walk on. Our environment is now the most toxic it has ever been. In human history. By every metric.

We are a species in the throes of extreme evolutionary change due to man-made conditions. Our bodies are attempting to adapt to a fast-changing climate beyond our control – environmentally, technologically, ideologically. The pace of life from the 1950s to 2010s has sped up more than any other time on Earth. Global warming is changing established seasons and weather patterns that our bodies and our food sources depend on. New viruses are crossing national and species barriers with greater frequency, disrupting health. Wars and terrorism are disrupting normal life in vast swathes of the world and skipping over national borders on planes. Medical abilities are enabling those who previously may have died in childhood to live longer, passing on greater genetic diversity. And we are being bombarded with information about all these things and more in a twenty-four hour stream of rolling news every time we pick up our smart phones. We are having to deal with these changes consciously and fast. But our bodies, our systems, are used to processing change slowly and unconsciously. As a result we are registering enormous amounts of instability, consciously and unconsciously, both as individuals and as a species. As our bodyminds try to process these unprecedented amounts of novel information that do not fit into our current intellectual or emotional framework (or paradigm). And so they respond to this unknown as a threat, registering pain, fear and trauma.

Scientists are now referring to our era as the Anthropocene, the first geological era ever shaped by a species, because the impact of our modern lives is affecting the very fossil record. According to Professor Jan Zalasiewicz, a geologist at the University of Leicester in an article for The Guardian, "The significance of the Anthropocene is that it sets a different trajectory for the Earth system, of which we of course are part."[18]

But those who stand to make a lot of money from the fuel we burn, the vehicles we drive, the chemicals we use and the medicines we take, prefer that our governments not focus too hard on their toxicity. They continue to sell the story with their advertising dollars that everything is fine: the good life is available to all at little cost, we've never had it so good. And why wouldn't they? They are not about to reveal damning data or change anything unless forced, because the way things are is working very well for them.

But they're not working for us as a species. People are not *just* physically sick, but struggling to stay alive. Scientists are now warning that the impact of climate change may be as large as economic recessions on rates of self-harm and suicide.[19] And air pollution has been shown to raise mental health issues in children.[20] Rates of suicide are up 25% since 1999 in the US.[21]

Our bodyminds – just like the rest of nature – are not used to this. This modern world that we are encouraged to consider normal, is anything but. It is new and fast-changing. That this would not have an impact on our exquisitely sensitive biological systems would be strange. They are, though we often forget it, a part of their natural environment. Our bodyminds are taking in this newness through every part, all the time: skin, hair, guts, ears, eyes, brains, lungs. What is out there becomes a part of us: chemicals, new viruses, radiation, electromagnetic pollution, microwaves…

What effect individual chemical factors are having, we are, to a degree, aware of because of the testing required by government agencies.

What cumulative effect these have, we truly have no idea.

Except we do.

Look at us. The effects are becoming apparent in the meteoric rise of allergies and autoimmune diseases, the rise in cancers and multiple chemical sensitivities. As one expert in the field of autoimmunity states, "The increasing incidence of Type 1 diabetes suggests a major environmental contribution, but the role of specific factors such as viruses remains controversial."[22]

Indeed some are accrediting this epidemic of chronic illness to a new virus such as Epstein-Barr or Lyme[23], sweeping out of control and weakening our immune systems. And it is entirely possible. New viruses are certainly sweeping through non-human populations unchecked, as ecosystems go out of balance. Whole species are dying off because of them including: bees, North American elm forests, thousand-year-old olive groves, two-thousand year-old kaori trees in New Zealand… We humans have certainly not been immune to new viruses in recent years. The world's attention, and media hysteria have followed one pandemic to the next – AIDS, SARS, Swine flu, Avian flu, Ebola, Zika virus. These illnesses have swept the world leaving death in their wake and Western medicine struggling to catch up.

But with chronic illness we cannot currently easily pinpoint the culprit. And perhaps, or rather probably, that is because there is not just one.

The fact that our individual, cultural and ecological systems are so unbalanced is contributing to our problems. Instability has become systemic in recent years. The stress levels of modern life have skyrocketed since the 2008 economic crash. People in every sector of society from students to business people, frontline teachers and health workers, to those reliant on government benefits have seen budgets slashed and the pressure to perform increase to unbearable levels. Greater economic and political instability, a loss of employment, longer work days, rising insurance costs, bankruptcy and repossession are daily worries for most. Austerity measures have come down hardest on those who receive government benefits, with child benefit payments cut, disability benefits being re-assessed and job seeker's benefit and single parent's payments under ever-tighter scrutiny and sanctions.

In the UK, for example, despite it being the third lowest level in Europe for persistent poverty, the Office for National Statistics found that between 2011-2014 more than a third of the UK population had lived in "relative poverty" earning below the poverty line (less than 60% of average pay) and that long-term poverty rates were worse for women.[24] The rise of zero hours contracts and the self-employed mean the loss of stable incomes, holidays and sick pay for vast swathes of the population. But not all.

This instability that is stressing and sickening a growing majority whilst killing off communities (the providers of informal care and support structures), is actively profiting those who are insulated from the shockwave by financial privilege and political power. Our increasing reliance on paid support services is further impoverishing those who are already ill and enriching those who are not: sickness is cementing social inequality.

The effects of economic and social inequality on our health are neither negligible nor imaginary: they have been known about since the 1970s. According to Richard Wilkinson and Kate Pickett in *The Spirit Level*, "More equal societies, such as Scandinavian nations, record lower levels of depression and higher levels of wellbeing overall, while depression is most common in highly unequal societies such as the United States and United Kingdom."

These stresses are on top of technological information overwhelm via the internet, rolling news of one disaster after another, electromagnetic pollution, sedentary lifestyles, processed food, increasing urbanisation, the raised terrorist threat, political instability and an ever-increasing disconnection from nature.

And that was before the typhoon of insanity that was 2016 onwards – Brexit, the Trump election and presidency, near constant terrorist attacks and mass shootings, the Grenfell tower fire, the renewed threat of nuclear war…

That is affecting us all, every man, woman, child.

But women seem to be hit first and hit hardest. And historically have been most ignored.

WHAT'S WRONG WITH WOMEN?

Women are half the world's population, yet they do two-thirds of the world's work, earn one-tenth of the world's income, and own less than one per cent of the world's property. They are among the poorest of the world's poor.
Barber Conable, former President of the World Bank

There is no good time to get sick. Especially if you're a woman.

Women are in the unique situation of being the majority of carers of the young, sick and aged in the world – and the totality of its life-bearers. But they have historically held far less political power or financial clout to make any systemic changes.

The strain on women within patriarchy is different. The nuclear family, an evolutionary new progeny of the Industrial Revolution, impinges far more on women's energy and resources. Women still live under political administrations that legislate against, or in ignorance of, their bodies (see the 2017 US Republican committee made up of thirteen men legislating on sweeping reforms to women's healthcare if you're in any doubt[25]) and much of their work, within a culture that encultures them not to assert or attend to their own needs. The World Health Organisation is clear on this when it unequivocally states:

Depression, anxiety, psychological distress, sexual violence, domestic violence and escalating rates of substance use affect women to a greater extent than men across different countries and different settings. Pressures created by their multiple roles, gender discrimination and associated factors of poverty, hunger, malnutrition, overwork, domestic violence and sexual abuse, combine to account for women's poor mental health. There is a positive relationship between the frequency and severity of such social factors and the frequency and severity of mental health problems in women.[26]

Women's sickness impacts the base level of society: housework (women still do over 60% more according to a 2016 survey by the UK Office of National Statistics[27]), family administration, carework, emotional labour… all of which *still* in the twenty-first century have been shown in study after study, the world over, to fall more heavily on women's shoulders. Often on top of a full-time job. Or three part-time shifts. Or single parenting.

"I don't have the luxury of falling apart," one mother said to me, faced with yet another health crisis in her family. And most of us don't. We are the links in the chain, the ones holding it all together for everyone else. And so we medicate and carry on. And on. And on. Even when we can't. Because we have to. Because there's no one lining up to take our places, to volunteer to do all this hard, undervalued work we do. We have to use every bit of our strength and unvalued life-force to keep the show on the road.

It is precisely *because* this gendered carework, as Vanessa Olorenshaw argues so powerfully in her book *Liberating Motherhood*, falls firmly outside of GDP and is done mainly in private that these stresses can be easily ignored and discounted. Because in patriarchy only what is done in public, only what is esteemed and paid, counts as *real work*. In short: traditionally men's work is work, and women's work isn't. So women keep expending their energy on things that don't officially count, as well as working harder than men for less pay in the outside world[28]... and then get the blame for being sick and tired... or told they're imagining it.

This dynamic is endemic to patriarchy: women are carrying the weight of the world on their shoulders and are crumbling under the strain as social, state and community supports are pulled from beneath them.

Despite the rising rates of autoimmune diseases, depression and anxiety in women, Western medicine is not focused on what it is about women's lives and the cultural environment that makes us sick. And it's not really looking into why modern medication doesn't help us to heal. Instead it's blaming the women who are sick for being sick in the first place. Or not believing that they even are.

Our culture is heavily invested in sustaining the lie that this unhealthy, unsustainable, toxic, man-made way of life is working. And it's reliant on our complicity to sustain it.

THE END OF BUSY/INESS AS USUAL

This disease of being "busy" (and let's call it what it is, the dis-ease of being busy, when we are never at ease) is spiritually destructive to our health and wellbeing.[29]
Omid Safi

What if there is something so fundamentally wrong with the world, the lives, and the way of being offered us, that withdrawal is the only sane response? Withdrawal, followed by a re-entry into a world, a life, and a way of being wholly different from the one left behind?
Charles Eisenstein, "Mutiny of the Soul".

Whilst the first question we raise when our bodies collapse is *what's wrong?* The second is usually *why now?*

Often illness feels like it comes out of the blue. We were just carrying on as normal. We might have got a bug or had a couple of extra stressors and then suddenly our bodies collapse for no good reason. It may be seen as a disproportionate response to us, to those around us, and is often treated as such by medical professionals. Especially in women.

So why now?

When we are constantly immersed in toxicity, as we are now, our bodies are constantly taking it on and trying to process it. When there is no time to rest, to recharge, to detox, when insanity and imbalance have become normality... then we have a problem. Then biological systems fail.

For women in our thirties to fifties we have probably been running on empty for too long. A woman's body and mind tend to be their most overstretched in her years of peak fertility and child-rearing, with internal resources stretched between menstruating, creating and growing new life, be it a career or a family or both, as well as a busy social life.

In our teens and twenties we're busy building a persona, and using all sorts of crutches in order to support this vision of ourselves that we are trying to project out into the world. We may set up bad habits and get away with them because of the combination of youth, fewer demands on us both emotionally and physically, and the fact that they are still reasonably new habits.

By the time we hit our thirties and beyond we are like over-stretched rubber bands, as Sara Heath so eloquently puts it in her chapter in *The Nine Degrees of Autism*: "When we are younger and more flexible, we all tend to be more 'elastic'. We can stretch quite thin to cope as a rubber band does, and then it returns to its normal size when the need to stretch has gone. The problem is when the rubber becomes old and worn or stretched too thin, then they snap. Mentally and physically this happens to us all, as well as metaphorically."[30]

Our bodies are made to be able to run on empty for short periods in order to survive. We are made to deal with stress, but when stress becomes long-term and inescapable it become toxic.

We may have had the warning signs of impending sickness, but not heeded them, or perhaps not been aware of them or told they were nothing to worry about.

In our culture of perfectionism the pressure is on from every side that everything has to be done to the highest of our ability. And it has to be done now. For women this pressure is even higher. We are expected to be super-human machines. And sexy too.

We're paying a high price, as women, to live in our modern world. And we're paying for it with our health, as well as our wallets.

And when we fail, we are treated not with compassionate care but with disbelief, condescension, antidepressants, anti-anxiety meds and painkillers.

Our bodies are displaying the symptoms of the truths we cannot tell. If our voices cannot be heard, then our bodies will tell the truth their way. Our bodies are protesting: they are calling time on this way of living, for an end to busyness as usual.

THE WHEEL OF DEATH

Roll up, roll up! Witness the incredible Wheel of Death!

We were drawn to it as children, to its flashing lights and bright colours, its entrancing music as it lifted off the ground, higher and higher, longing for the day that we were old enough to ride it.

The wheel was fun at first – education, job, money, housing, kids, travel...

The sense of freedom and exhilaration as we started spinning, the rush of adrenaline as we took off defying gravity. *Look at us go!* we screamed in excitement.

Scream if you want to go faster! they replied.

We screamed, throwing our heads back laughing, feeling like masters of the universe. The wheel went higher and higher, faster and faster. Fun began to morph into fear. We saw the ground blurring beneath us.

We scream.

There is no way off now. The safety belts no longer feel there for our safety, they're digging in, restraining us: keeping us on a ride we no longer want to be on.

We scream more.

We go faster.

We scream again. And again. And again.

For it to stop.

This has become the Wheel of Death for real. Our bodies are barely able to take the strain of the forces upon them – heads spinning, noses bleeding, vomiting, passing out.

Screaming.

Screaming.

Some wriggle free, some fall out.

Down...

Down...

Down...

They fall. The rest of us watch. Barely able to focus. Helpless. Wondering what will happen to those who fall.

Is this our fate? Is there life beyond the wheel? Are we helpless or just disorientated? How can we slow it down and see? Or do we have to jump and trust?

RECLAIMING THE HEALING ARTS

If you want to feel better, make something. Make anything.
All creativity aligns us with creation itself, the source of all healing.
Martha Beck

At the end of every chapter there are Medicine Questions and Healing Arts exercises to help integrate what you have read. The intention of these is to create an immersive, multi-sensory, somatic experience, much as the writing of this book has been for me. I wholeheartedly recommend that you read through these sections, even if you do not have time to do them right away, as often the exercises dive deeper into the material.

These sections are most definitely not just an optional extra if you are wanting to embody your healing. The Western world tends to keep us in our heads, stuck in the fear-driven hamster-wheel of the mind that we try to escape from through dissociative practices. Reading can become another dissociative practice that keeps us stuck in our minds. We can believe that if we just read the book and understand the issue logically then we've done the work. Take it from one who has spent a lifetime doing that!

Without the tools to navigate this process we can feel scared, lost and alone. Illness brings us back into the physical reality of our bodies whilst simultaneously uncovering the inner parts of ourselves that we prefer to keep hidden. Our bodies are bringing up the raw material we need to work with in order to heal, but often we do not know what to do with it. So we try to shut it down.

In the past, and in other cultures, there has been a deep connection between the role of artist and healer.[31] Creative practices help us to move from understanding healing as a cure that comes from outside of ourselves, to knowing healing as an ongoing process of inner and outer transformation and self-realisation that we can actively engage with. It helps us to listen more deeply to our bodyminds, to honour their experiences as rich and valid material for our creative practice and to connect directly to the source of healing and creativity, which is one and the same.

Metaphor, image, emotion are the language of the unconscious mind, body and soul. Finding the words and images to express the struggling, bubbling, chaotic realms within can be both inherently calming and soothing, as well as revealing of insights into the body and unconscious mind in unforeseen ways that we are then able to make changes to.

I am not a trained therapist in any discipline, but have borrowed from a lot of different therapeutic traditions, using my creativity to work through my mental and physical health journey and shed light on the healing process. Painting, drawing, writing, movement, clay work and making patterns with found objects have given me expression when I have felt wordless and alone. They have engaged my bodymind when it felt completely stuck and have helped me to begin the process of reaching out – for help, support, treatment and companionship.

The WORD+image process I have developed – part art therapy, part soul journey – which I will touch on in these exercise, has become an integral part of my own practice. In essence it looks a little like art journaling though with the emphasis on the inner process rather than creating a work of art for show – the focus is on expressing inner states and thoughts through a combination of words and images.

Please know that you don't need to be an artist to try any of these exercises. They are not about creating a beautiful end-product for show, but a way of mapping our messy inner processes in a way that makes them visible to us, encouraging healthy self-expression of our inner realities. Nor do you need a whole heap of expensive artist materials. Most exercises can be done with what you will find around your home: an unruled journal, sketchbook or sheets of plain paper, a pencil, some coloured markers, and perhaps some old magazines, scissors and glue. My creative motto always is *Do What You Can, With What You Have, Where You Are*. So be brave, pick a creative exercise that excites or intrigues you, read through the instructions, and dive into it. Feel free to adapt it and make it your own. Have fun reclaiming the healing arts for yourself, or with your best friend, kids or women's circle. Remember, especially if you are a working artist, that these are healing exercises for yourself, please do not put any pressure on yourself to share the results of them with anyone. If you do want to share them, choose your audience with care and wisdom and deep self-love: this is vulnerable work, and you, love, deserve to feel safe as you do it courageously.

MEDICINE QUESTIONS

Asking the proper question is the central action of transformation…
Questions are the keys that cause the secret doors of the psyche to
swing open.
Clarissa Pinkola Estés, *Women Who Run With the Wolves*

Questions are a cornerstone of my work, as those who have read my other books can attest. I get so much feedback on the importance of the questions in my books in helping to prompt the inner journeys of my readers.

My personal journals and writing notebooks are filled with questions. Finding the right question, I have discovered, is often more important than finding the right answer. Naming has power. The right question often lifts the veil on our invisible assumptions and opens the door to healing: our minds become receptive to new channels of information. Resources and possibilities that we may previously have overlooked seem to be drawn to us as if by magic. It seems that we naturally begin to live into the answers once the right question has been posed.

This all sounds so exciting, right? But healing tends to require asking uncomfortable questions. The questions we have avoided. The questions we have evaded. The questions we would rather silence.

There are lots of questions here. Please don't be overwhelmed by them. Each reader will have different needs and challenges. As you run your eye over them see which questions you are drawn to, and which you want to immediately avoid. Both, I would suggest, hold medicine for you. Those that do not interest you, pass them on by for now. They may be of use at another time, or to another woman. They may well help you formulate your own questions.

You might want to work through these questions yourself – either in your journal, in meditation or in discussion with a friend, counsellor or therapist, or with other women in your own Medicine Woman circle, red tent, book club or women's group.

Please remember there are no 'right' answers. Answer from your guts rather than from your head, from intuition and body memory not logic. Pay close attention. Bring yourself to these questions with radical honesty, and listen to yourself as you respond, trying to feel into your body as you do. Where there is no answer, where there are no words, simply allow the question into your body and sit with it. Do any images appear, however nonsensical they might seem? Do you feel a pain or tension when you consider a question? Is there a flash of anger or sadness? Can you follow that sensation and stay with it? Where does it take you?

It will bring you back, back to yourself, my love.

Childhood Experiences of Sickness

What experiences of illness did you have as a child?

Do you have any photographs of your illnesses or recovery? Can you find them and reconnect visually and emotionally with that child?

What did you learn about what being sick meant from influential adults as you grew up?

How were you cared for?

What experiences did you have of doctors and medicine when you were growing up?

Did any of your close family suffer from a major illness during your childhood? How was this explained to you? What was the result of it? How did you react? Do you have any photographs of this time? Can you look them out in order to reconnect visually and emotionally with the people then, and who they are now?

What was your interpretation of why illness happened as a child? Did you feel any guilt, fear or sadness? How were you helped to process these feelings? What feelings do you still hold about your childhood experiences? Has it informed your adult experience of sickness? Can you talk this through with those you went through it with to hear other perspectives or more details that may have been hidden from you as a child?

How do you respond to the illness of others today?

Have you had to play the role of carer to others? What impact has this had on you physically, mentally and emotionally? Did you have support in this caring role? Did you feel valued in it?

How has caring for others impacted how you take care of yourself?

Your Sense of Health

What does wellness or health mean to you? Are they the same thing?

How would you describe your sense of wellness at the moment? How frequently are you ill? How do you feel about this?

Can you draw, write or describe aloud how it feels to live in your body right now? Was it always like this? Can you identify when it changed?

What do you have to do to be well/healthy? How does your lifestyle currently support your wellness?

Do you think your sickness is your fault? Do you feel shame or guilt connected to it?

What parts of your bodymind are dominating your attention right now?

What parts of your bodymind are you consciously or unconsciously ignoring?

Health Check

In the following exercise I suggest a comprehensive self health check. In it you list all your physical, mental and emotional symptoms in a way that works best for you. Later exercises in the book will come back to this activity and add to it, so I do recommend doing it.

You may like to do this in a hand-drawn table in your journal, or perhaps you would prefer to create an Excel spreadsheet on your computer. It could also be done as a spider chart or mind map with lots of colours and images. I have given an example over the page.

This exercise works particularly well for visual learners, but is a great tool for everyone, as it means that you have to make visible all the symptoms you are dealing with. This helps you to move out of denial, and see how long things have been bothering you, and how the treatments you are using are working. It is also a great tool to take with you to your doctor or other healing ally*, so that they have a potted medical history at a glance.

1. First list each of your main physical or emotional symptoms.

2. Under this put another row noting when the symptoms started.

3. Next, how frequently (and severely) you get these symptoms. Note down any seasonal, cyclical or other connections (for example do you always get a headache after being in bright sunshine, during the winter or after eating chocolate?)

4. In another row, mark down if it has been formally diagnosed, if so when and what the diagnosis was. If you don't have a diagnosis put a question mark in the box, or what you suspect it might be.

5. In the next row, note if there is a family history of this condition.

6. In the next row, note down if you are currently receiving any treatment (including self-care) for it and what this treatment is.

7. Leave a spare couple of rows at the end for a later exercise.

SYMPTOM	*Headaches with nausea and exhaustion*
FIRST STARTED	*Age 15*
FREQUENCY	*Monthly – usually in the week before my period, after eating chocolate, flashing lights.*
FAMILY HISTORY	*Yes, mother*
DIAGNOSIS, DIAGNOSED BY	*Migraine (classic) – Dr Alvarez, 1996*
TREATMENT	*Paracetamol* *Avoiding food triggers*
RESULTS	*Works if taken immediately at onset.* *Effective, but hard when premenstrual.*

Your Journey So Far

How can you creatively express your inner journey of sickness and your interactions with the medical profession? How have these intersected? Where have they diverged? You may choose to use words, collage, painting, drawing, dance or drama to share the high and low points of this experience so far.

The Wheel of Death

How resonant was this metaphor for you? Can you remember when you first stepped onto the wheel, and how you were feeling? Have you managed to get off it yet?

Can you create an image of what the wheel looks like or feels like to you?

The Mask

What is the mask that you present to the world? When and where did you learn to wear it? Were you given it by someone? How much energy and effort does it take to sustain this mask? What lies beneath this mask? Who has seen beneath it? How do you feel about this?

Find a photograph of yourself where the mask is fully intact, a moment when you were projecting the image of "fine" or even "successful"? How do you feel about this image? How were you feeling underneath at the time? Who approved of this image? How did that make you feel?

Find an image of yourself without the mask. How does this image make you feel? What were you told about it? How did that make you feel?

Can you draw, collage or take a photographic image to represent yourself and the mask you wear? Can you find a way of visually revealing what lies beneath? Perhaps you would like to make a mask of your own face or purchase a papier mâché one from a craft store and decorate it. You might choose to paint your own face with face paints, perhaps half of it masked, and half of it revealing what lies underneath. Take a photograph of yourself masked/unmasked, stick it into your journal, and use half of the page to write what it feels like to wear a mask, and half to reflect on how it feels to take it off.

DIAGNOSIS

This was the way medicine worked: tests told you what was wrong,
and doctors told you how to fix it.[32]
Meghan O'Rourke

The meaning of the word 'diagnosis' comes from the Greek, *gnosis* – 'knowledge' and *dia* – 'apart'. Taken together they mean "to distinguish or discern". The Merriam Webster dictionary defines it as "the art or act of identifying a disease from its signs and symptoms." Medical diagnosis holds tremendous power within our culture.

Like the Hogwarts sorting hat, a medical diagnosis can help you find which box you best fit within, so that you can find the medicine or treatment options most likely to help your condition.

This official naming gives form to the intangible: translating our lived experience into terms that our culture recognises, interpreting your physical symptoms, energy levels and behaviours into something universally comprehensible, which can then be cured, treated or managed. It also helps the individual to access services, supports and social understanding. More than just a personal identification of what ails you, a diagnosis is a key in the door to the System. It doesn't matter what you may privately think, believe, know or say about the health of your own bodymind. It doesn't matter your evidence, experience or certainty. If it doesn't come from an approved physician, given in medical terms, it is not real to the System.

THE JOURNEY TO KNOWLEDGE

We can't name our sickness, nor do we know what our medicine could be [...] Through the symptoms in our bodies and in our families she speaks of what is out of balance. She will tell us the name of our illness and the name of our medicine. But [...] we have to ask the right questions over and over[...] We have to listen to the answers and then take responsibility to act.
Starhawk and Hilary Valentine, *The Twelve Wild Swans*

Most of the time the path to diagnosis starts as a personal journey. We get vague hints that something might be wrong in our bodies – the strange rash, the aching head, the unexplained tiredness, the raised temperature, the worry of this, the wondering about that. Then the realisation that this might be a 'thing' but an uncertainty about what this thing is or how serious it might be. This tends to lead us to Google searches, books and asking friends all the while trying to discern the pattern of these symptoms for ourselves, trying to crack their code. For many this is an anxious time: knowing something is wrong, but not knowing what or how serious it is. Many of us tend to swing between denial, "It's nothing, it'll go away if I ignore it" to panic, "It's cancer and I'm going to die" as we scroll through grotesque images and worst-case scenarios in our heads and on our computer screens.

If we recognise the symptoms from previous experience with friends or family, we may feel empowered to take action ourselves without involving medical professionals. Or we might know which healing ally to seek out. This experience of self-diagnosis and self-treatment, when we have certainty and know what response is required, is usually an empowering one. Even if it necessitates a quick trip to a doctor, we tend to receive fast diagnosis and treatment.

Certainty is by no means guaranteed when we decide to follow the path of formal diagnosis. There are times when the experts cannot be certain or contradict each other. There are occasions when multiple conditions are diagnosed. Or when your symptoms do not correlate with an existing condition which is currently understood in our culture, at this point in history or part of the world. Then there are times when the professionals are unable to interpret the results they find, cannot find enough evidence or do not do the right combination of tests at the right time. Times when the doctor's prejudices blind them to your reality. In these cases, diagnosis becomes less definitive or satisfying. This, sadly, is what many women experience in their journey of sickness: a lack of belief in their suffering and a lack of clear cut answers, despite dedicating themselves to a search for them.

Many chronic conditions entail a lengthy journey to specialist after specialist, with many stop-gap diagnoses which don't quite fit. There may be a long wait on a public health waiting list, or the struggle to find the funds for a private diagnosis. The whole experience can feel extremely disempowering.

For many of us this part of the journey is simply too much to bear. We give up before we even start, avoiding doctors altogether. Or we may give up several years down the line having run out of funds, energy or motivation. And we endeavour once more to push our suffering aside, as we have been told, and get on with life as best we can.

For some of us the strength to pursue our own diagnosis may only come when someone we love gets sick and the Medicine Woman within us emerges. She who will do whatever it takes to protect her beloved child. She who will turn over every stone until answers are found to heal her.

Often it is only in the deep commitment that our daughters will not suffer as we have, that we speak up, that we pursue our own diagnosis. We insist that the nameless finally be named. Only then do we change the story of female silence. And only then can we look again with new compassion at our sisters, mothers and grandmothers, at the burden they carried that went unseen, untreated or mistreated. For those that are still alive, they get the gift of seeing their children and grandchildren receive opportunities and treatments that were not open to them: they get to see the story change. And perhaps, if they are willing, they can receive the recognition – in the form of acknowledgement, diagnosis and support for what they have suffered all these years. In this way we heal up and down the family line.

We may. Or we may receive condemnation for naming what had been left purposely unsaid, for exposing what had been left hidden. When we break the conspiracy of silence that has denied our female pain, we play with fire: a fire that can hurt or heal.

The thing that shocked me more than anything else was the loss of friends and family who, to this day, have not spoken to me since my diagnosis. People I thought were always going to be there for me, weren't. That hurt more than the diagnoses themselves. I do know that some of them think that I am 'putting this on to gain attention' and others think I'm downright lying about my test results and diagnoses.

HEATHER

Diagnosis can create a path through the wilderness, a way back home, a parting of clouds and seeing of the light. It can be a ten-thousand-piece puzzle done without the lid of the box or untangling a ball of wool that has been cut at multiple points. It can be a bolt from the blue. Or it might be a sentence emerging from the silence – a life sentence, a death sentence. When we start out on the path we do not know. But the fear of what might be can hold us back, just as a longing for healing can propel us forwards.

With diagnosis tends to come a whole raft of emotions: relief, validation, vilification, a feeling of finally being seen, heard and believed, as well as grief, anger, denial, overwhelm, powerlessness, despair, sadness, numbness, frustration at the time taken, the opportunities for healing lost, the lack of services and support available. There can be a feeling of tremendous isolation from loved ones, a sense of alienation of being different from others, being alone in this situation, misunderstood or abandoned. There can be guilt at being ill, at the burden we feel we are or will be to our loved ones or at the expense it will entail.

How do we know in advance what diagnosis will bring for us or our families? In truth we cannot. It is an act of great courage and vulnerability. We hope that it will bring healing, but we do not know for sure. We can stack the odds in our favour and control the process as best we can. We can ask for recommendations of experienced or like-minded physicians, look for second opinions, seek support from those who have walked this path before us. We can do our research, reading up on the condition and its treatments, making informed decisions. But after that, either we choose knowledge, or we do not.

WOMEN AND DIAGNOSIS

Women struggle to get their needs met by doctors because the profession is overwhelmingly male. [...] There is not a single female MP who hasn't told me at some point they felt patronised and diminished whilst trying to access health treatments. [If] female MPs, who were pushy, articulate, good-at-looking-after-ourselves kinds of women, had problems, then it suggested there was a wider issue.[33]
**Jackie Doyle-Price, minister for mental health,
The Guardian, June 2018.**

For many women, diagnosis, and the path that leads to it, is a deeply problematic part of Western medicine. Pursuing diagnosis can be a crash course in self-esteem and advocacy, often at one of the most vulnerable and lowest points of a woman's life, when she is scared and in pain.

Many women have experienced personal and family histories of physical, sexual or emotional abuse; lack of consent; loss of independence or identity; mismanagement, disbelief or cruelty at the hands of authorities. If we have, then medical assessment and treatment can be tinged with a feeling of profound powerlessness, underlaid by layers of trauma.

Those who have not experienced these issues firsthand will have heard stories and learned their lessons of how women have been mistreated by the System. It is little wonder that most women turn first not to their family doctor, but to Dr Google to figure out what is wrong with them.

....

*I stumbled accidentally upon my 'diagnosis' via Dr Google. I found a support group full of people who had exactly the same symptoms. Backing up this support group was a pile of scientific research going back to the 1960s/70s, and two current medical doctors who were actively working in the field, one in America and one in Japan.
But despite all this research, and despite the growing community of sufferers, GPs and dermatologists were in denial of the diagnosis. So my diagnosis was personal, linked to a community of other sufferers, and this is how I supported myself through the process of healing – by trial, error, lots of experimentation, research and intuition.*

It was a relief to find an explanation because I'd been struggling with worsening symptoms of all sorts for years, and no doctor ever gave me any indication that the drugs I was taking were the problem. I fought it in some sense, in that I kept reading (through case studies and connections to other sufferers) the healing time was a minimum of a year, more like three. I was sure I could heal myself much quicker, of course!

It helped enormously having that personal diagnosis because it gave me a definite plan of action, and it armed me with knowledge to approach my doctors for the support that was within their remit to give (not much, but I did at least get some [government sickness benefit] through it). It also helped me to show my family what I was doing and why – because they all thought I was crazy denying conventional medical help. Nobody had heard of iatrogenicity. Everyone who met me thought I was dying. Even my landlord was shocked at how quickly I'd gone downhill and offered some free homeopathy sessions. Without my diagnosis, I'd have kept going around in circles and ultimately ended up worsening my health instead of climbing out of the pit.

For a long time I kept referring to myself as ill, and when I started to get better, I'd say "when I was really ill". In the last year I've learned to say "healing crisis" instead, which is much more accurate. I was ill before – chronically ill in numerous ways, and then I started to heal myself. But I got much worse before I got better.

ZOË

There is a growing cultural shift in women's scepticism towards diagnosis and health authorities that is showing up in a reluctance to engage with medical services. In the UK attendance at cervical smear tests is at a twenty-year low with 1.27 million missed appointments in the 2016-17 period.[34] UK uptake in mammogram screening is at its lowest level in a decade.[35] Health authorities are struggling to reach targets for flu vaccination uptake in pregnant women, HPV in teen girls, multiple vaccines in babies.[36] This is despite increased public education and advertising campaigns, and all these procedures being completely free of charge.

Are women losing faith in Western medicine's ability to diagnose them correctly and keep them healthy?

DIAGNOSIS: A CULTURAL FRAMEWORK

My diagnosis isn't about sinking into defeatism. My diagnosis is about helping me love the bits of myself that I've always found confusing. My symptoms don't define me, but my coping mechanisms do.[37]
Anna Hart

In the medical world, diagnoses are often treated as definitive definitions of reality, rather than as an individual's interpretation using limited tests at a distinct point in time. Interpretations do and have shifted throughout history. They are as much a reflection of our cultural understanding of what disease is and what it means to be human *at this very moment in history*, as they are an objective labelling of the body.

In each era some sicknesses come with a strong stigma – plague and leprosy in the Middle Ages, AIDS in the 1980s, Ebola today. Some become non-existent when cultural expectations shift – note the ubiquity of hysteria in Victorian times, versus its virtual oblivion today, or the total disappearance of Asperger Syndrome from US psychiatric labelling in 2013. So, when we take on a label, we also take on what that label means in and to our culture, and the treatment – medical and social – that goes along with it. We take the prejudices and the limitations into our bodyminds and inhabit them in the eyes of others: we can become shaped by the label that is put on us.

Western medical science tends to focus on what it *does* know, not all the grey areas which it has not mapped out. And in our desire for the ultimate truth of a "gold-plated" diagnosis and to be able to fully believe in the expertise of those we have trusted, often we forget our own cultural limitations. Most of us are blind to the current paradigm: the mindset that shapes our knowing and that of our medical professionals. We forget, or are encouraged not to know, that just as there are many ways of knowing, and many languages to speak of knowledge in, there are also many ways of understanding sickness and many paths to healing.

The same condition can be named in many different ways: what one expert calls clinical depression, another calls possession by devils, another sees the isolation from community, systemic exhaustion or simply the need to pull oneself together. For a doctor of Chinese medicine depression might come about due to a blockage of chi (life-force energy), for a Western doctor it is due to low levels of serotonin, for a psychotherapist it might be patterns of negative thinking or suppressed childhood trauma, in New Age healing it is resonating at a lower level of consciousness and a need to ground your energy. Such different interpretations for the same set of symptoms. And such different treatments ranging from herbs and needles, to daily SSRI medication, to talking and painting, to exorcism or "cheer up and get on with it", to consciousness raising retreats and walks in nature. Each naming comes from a different perspective and methodology. Each is the expression of a particular paradigm, a fundamental way of understanding the body and mind. Each holds within it a distinct seed of treatment, a unique set of priorities and protocols.

But at present each exists in a separate bubble. Each holds his dogma as the one and only truth. And often raises doubts about the others' validity or expertise. And we, the sick, are left not knowing where to turn or who to trust.

PROGNOSIS

It is not just our present or past which is mapped by a diagnosis, but our future too. When we receive a diagnosis we are expected to accept the story about what is 'wrong' and why, which medicine will be required to make us better and what the story of treatment will be. With the label given by diagnosis comes the narrative of the illness – the prognosis, meaning "knowing before". We learn what our lives will look like, what ending to anticipate, how long the telling of it will last.

I have avoided pursuing a full 'diagnosis' or 'labelling' because I don't trust most of the medical treatments. I feel like they would just try and give me a pill to deal with it, and I don't want that for myself.
DIANA

When we receive a diagnosis of chronic or life-threatening illness within Western medicine, it may feel as though our own biography, life and choices have been pushed aside, or even erased, and the medical story placed on top, subsuming our lives and identities. Our days become crowded with hospital visits, medical apparatus and time marked by the taking of different coloured tablets. We may feel powerless, surrendered to the medical behemoth that consumes us whole, but which, we are told, holds in its hands our only hope of survival.

After diagnosis often comes the battle, both internal and external, not to be defined solely by the label we have been given. We struggle to have our suffering fully acknowledged and treated, but our sickness seen simply as a part of our humanity. It may define many aspects of our daily life, may create all sorts of limitations, but it is not *all* we are. We are not *just* our conditions.

With acute illnesses we tend to say, "I have the flu" – so that the disease is seen as separate to the person, who retains primacy and agency. Whereas with many chronic conditions, especially ones originating in the brain, we say "She is bipolar", or "He is autistic". For some, this way of defining the person through the condition is key – the two are so strongly intertwined in their expression that the individual cannot be experienced except through the lens of the condition. But the issue is that for many this lens can create expectations, can create a sense of disability, limitation or victimisation: the whole person is obscured behind the condition. This loss of identity, loss of personhood and agency is one of the greatest issues of the medicalisation of illness (we will go into this in more detail in a later chapter) and the way that we treat sick people in our culture as 'less than' or 'other'. This innate disempowerment at the heart of how diagnosis and healing are approached within the Western medical paradigm are a major part of why I believe women so often avoid diagnosis and medical intervention: women are fed up of being labelled and limited by our culture. We just want to be free to be seen as ourselves.

After years of all kinds of therapy, I turned into a high-functioning anx-ious, with several OCDs. At 24 I was also diagnosed with fibromyalgia. For years, I accepted what life had to offer (under these labels and conventional therapy and medicines). When my daughter was born (after a complicated pregnancy which ended with a pre-eclampsia) my mindset changed and I started looking for new answers: naturopathic medicine, clinical hypnosis, mind control, neurofeedback, finding my 'calling' and a divorce helped a lot.
I am not a different person but I live a different life, accepting these are my challenges and that I have to get the most out of life each and every day.
PATRICIA

So, is diagnosis and labelling a good thing, or something we should avoid? For many the fear of *what if* – the fear of stigma, the fear of losing control of one's own body, mind or identity to the System – is greater than the desire to heal or find support. But I fully believe that diagnosis and labelling, if done in an empowering manner by a compassionate and experienced healing ally, can help us find an-swers, understand the unique needs of our bodyminds more clearly and access the supports and treatments that we need to live healthier, happier lives. To begin to heal we must understand the current state of the body accurately. And we must treat it based on evidence, not guesswork.

I believe that diagnosis should never be the end of the story, but the beginning of a new chapter. It does not have to define how our story turns out, but it helps us to know where we're starting from.

So many hold back at the threshold. Because being labelled sick is shameful or a threat to the lives they do not want to lose. Because they fear the treatment that it will entail, the prognosis that will dis-empower them. And so they suffer in silence. Unseen, unsupported, uncared for. Alone.

THE MAKING REAL OF SICKNESS

Illness weaves through our lives with surprising regularity. It is no less central to the human condition than sexuality is, though we hardly give it the same attention.
Kat Duff, *The Alchemy of Illness*

If we are sick, but are undiagnosed, are we really sick? Is our sickness an empirical reality if we don't make a fuss? If we chose not to label it, does it exist? If we can paper a smile over our suffering, are we actually okay?

Until we are diagnosed we are often blamed for our struggles. Until it is formally recognised our *lived reality* is not recognised as *reality*. Undiagnosed conditions tend to lead to more ill health: a whole host of complications, and worse long-term prognoses. The longer we go undiagnosed and untreated, the sicker we tend to get: denial and avoidance are almost never the best medicine.

But for many of us this choice is still preferable to the fuss, the fear, the strain and the reality of diagnosis. Because often the 'making real' of our illness is the coming to pass of our darkest fears. It may awaken memories of loved ones who suffered. It may destroy our self-image as powerful, capable women. It may require that we come out as sick to a world that is intolerant or victimising of illness and disability.

. . . .

My illnesses are part of me. They are in me. They are me. My physical problems are part of my make-up, that is clear. They are the parts people accept, my parents and sibling accept, the parts people can talk about. The mental issues, however, are what define me. But they are put under the carpet and are never talked about. Except between my husband and I. I've recently mentioned snippets to my children as I have seen stress and anxiety issues in them, and I don't want it to be taboo. I want to break the cycle. I want them to feel it's okay, they are normal, it's nothing to be ashamed of. When I was diagnosed with a large ovarian cyst I needed it to be taken out right away. It shouldn't be there, I felt it was foreign. It wasn't there from the beginning. But everything else must have been there. I was a 'difficult' baby, stopped

my mother from having anymore. I was always clingy and needy, so my
anxiety must have always been there. My mother has extreme anxiety
and is a worrier but even now in her eighties she would never admit it.
In her eyes, only I have the problem.
JOANNE

If doctors are there to help us, why is it that many women are scared of, traumatised by and resistant to interactions with them? Why do we instinctively resist what might make us better?

I believe it is not just our own internal fears of sickness and death, nor our fear of social reactions – though they are significant. It is that the medical profession, for many of us, especially women, does not represent compassion and healing, but judgement and fear.

To understand this more clearly, we need to examine what passes for healing and medicine within the dominant culture, and examine why it is so problematic, especially for women and other groups that have been othered.

There is a politics to medicine. There is an economics. There is a history. There is a culture. But these tend to be overlooked.

In the next part of the book we will speak the unspoken, lifting the lid on why Western medical approaches can often be challenging for women. Together we will explore the power imbalance within it, and make visible some of the prejudices, limitations and history of the System we inhabit, on our way to discovering how we can choose to heal at last.

SCARED

Who can I trust to interpret my body?

Who can I trust to read it as holy scripture?

I am scared.

This fear is as infectious as any disease. The doctors shrink from it, when they see its symptoms in me: the dripping eyes, the reddening face, the tremor in the voice, the caught breath in the throat.

What if I am too scared to rise above it?

What if I am too scared to walk into his room, to put myself in his hands?

What if I am dying?

What if he thinks I'm crazy?

Will I be believed?

This is the question that always echoes.

I am scared that it will be all my fault – that I came too soon, or not early enough, that I should have noticed this, or need to learn to ignore that. That I am too sensitive. That it's all in my head.

This interaction between us, I never realised how intimate it was.

I am expected to offer up my body, my fluids, open my legs, pull down my top, bear my heart, open my mouth wide, tell you my most embarrassing secrets. What will you do with this evidence of me? Will you be gentle? Will you care? Will you see what I need you to?

I feel scared that I will be judged. That this thing that is wrong is not wrong at all – and that I am wrong for thinking it is.

I am scared that wheels will be set in motion that I cannot control. Wheels that will order my life. Will take charge. Of my body. My children. My world.

Do you know the power you hold?

Do you know how scared I am?

For you I am just a name on a long to-do list of today.
Just another bulging file of notes on your trolley.
Just another body on your bed.
To me it is everything.
This is my life, which I offer up to you.

Can I trust you with it?

MEDICINE QUESTIONS

Your Journey to Diagnosis

How do you know whether to trust a healthcare professional? How have your previous experiences with medical professionals influenced this?

How important is it that you receive an official diagnosis?

What does diagnosis mean to you emotionally?

Is official diagnosis the only way you felt that your suffering would be taken seriously? Is it the only way to access care, support or treatment?

Have you had to push or fight for diagnosis or was it a shock?

What have you found healing or empowering about receiving a diagnosis?

What have you found disempowering or traumatic about receiving a diagnosis?

Do you trust the diagnosis you have received? Why?

To what extent do you feel defined by your diagnosis today? Has this changed since your initial diagnosis?

Which parts of it accurately reflect your inner experience of the condition and which don't?

To what extent is your diagnosis understood by yourself/your healing allies/your community/the world in general?

Are you aware of how your diagnosis might be different in other cultures or times in history? Are you aware of how it might have been treated differently?

How do you feel you are perceived by others because of your condition? How much does this matter to you?

Beyond Diagnosis

What would you like people to know about the inner experience of your illness? What are the scariest parts? What are the most painful parts? What are the invisible aspects? What impacts your daily life the most and how? Does your illness come with any special abilities or has it changed your life in a way that is positive? You may want to create a collage, mind map or art journal a piece on your diagnosis – use half of the page to express society's perception of your condition and the other half to express your inner experience.

How might you use your own experience to help inform or educate others? These might include: those who have just been diagnosed, trainee medics, therapists, school children, parents, the community at large... You might choose to write a blog post, make a meme, create a graphic novel, poster or comic strip, write a poem, a play or a video diary... and then share it!

Untangling the Threads

The aim of this book is to help you to begin to untangle the threads of your illness, so that you can understand what it is you are actually dealing with.

Often the most overwhelming part of illness is the fact that there is not just one thing wrong but a tangle of different things: physical, mental, emotional, environmental and perhaps spiritual. The Western medical approach is to take each main physical symptom and treat it whilst ignoring all the other elements. In the previous exercise you listed the symptoms you are experiencing. In this one, we are exploring the factors underpinning your body and life that are influencing you right now. Western medicine may be able to help you deal with some parts, holistic medicine with others, self-care and education may fill the other needs.

Take a little time to write some notes on each of the following. Or alternatively you might want to do it as a spider diagram with each of the main areas in your life (the key people, the current situations) each as a separate branch, with the main issues branching out from each:

⬤ *What is currently stressing me about my home-life is...*

⬤ *What is currently stressing me about my work-life is...*

⬤ *What is currently stressing me about my sex-life is...*

- ⓘ *World events that are on my mind are…*

- ⓘ *I am currently grieving…*

- ⓘ *What I am struggling to express is…*

- ⓘ *My relationship with my parent(s) is…*

- ⓘ *My relationship with… (do this for each of your children, close friends, healing allies, community members)*

- ⓘ *The way I currently feel about myself is…*

- ⓘ *The most traumatic event in the past year was… I dealt with it by…*

- ⓘ *The most traumatic event in my adulthood was… I dealt with it by…*

- ⓘ *The most traumatic event in my childhood was… I dealt with it by…*

- ⓘ *Compared to usual my energy levels are…*

- ⓘ *My relationship to food is…*

- ⓘ *My relationship to exercise is…*

- ⓘ *I feel helpless in/with/about…*

Beyond Your Culture

Are you aware of how your diagnosis might be different in other cultures or times in history? Are you aware of how it might have been treated differently? Go online or look out some books on your condition or medical history. Create a timeline or perhaps a world map, or a collage incorporating the different names of your condition, the roots of these words, the believed cures. Which of these had you been aware of before? Do any give you further insight into your condition or possible ways to heal it or understand it better?

WHAT'S WRONG WITH WESTERN MEDICINE?

*Pathology is not merely something that is cured by well-meaning profes-
sionals and therapeutic technologies. This assumes the wellness of the
helper and sickness of the patient... It is widely acknowledged that the
therapeutic system itself is often pathological.*
Shaun McNiff, *Art as Medicine*

*The aim of medicine is to prevent disease and prolong life, the ideal of
medicine is to eliminate the need of a physician.*
William J. Mayo, one of the founders of the Mayo Clinic, the first and largest integrated, not-for-profit medical group practice in the world.

Medicine evolved alongside humanity, arising from the basic need
to help people who were suffering. Its job: to figure out what ails us
and try to make us better. This is still at the heart of medicine today.
However, throughout history other things have become conjoined to
medicine and doctoring within the Western scientific tradition, often
clouding its original purpose. Other parts have been surgically removed, causing long-term human trauma as standard. It is these parts
that I wish to examine here in a critical analysis of a System that has
been very good at penning its own glorification, championing its own
advances and memorialising its own heroes, whilst ignoring or negat-
ing the extensive dark side that has been systematically imposed on
patients, practitioners and our culture for centuries.

I am aware that following some of these threads may be painful for many readers. For others they may be familiar knowledge. I hesitate to plunge deep into the darkness, to rehash history, to unsettle the ghosts of the past that still haunt the present. I, too, want to get straight to the heart of healing. But I feel it would be remiss to omit what led us to where we are now. To be able to give voice to past trauma – individual or collective – is a key part of our healing. Whitewashing the past will not help us to make a brighter future. Nor will being unaware of it.

For many of us our aversion to medicine as it is now is unconscious, and so our resistance to doctors or diagnosis can seem irrational. We can berate ourselves for our fear, chide ourselves for our silliness when we get upset at being dismissed, ignored, talked over or treated without consent.

I want, I need, to show you that how you feel is not trivial. Not silly. Not insignificant. It is based on firm evidence, on obscured historical roots deeply felt but not overtly spoken of. I want to show you that the way you are treated by the medical system is not happenstance. I need to pull the curtain back on the way that medicine, hospitals and doctoring as we know them today have evolved, so that we can understand that they are not the *only* way to heal, nor necessarily the *healthiest* way to heal for us as women. But nor are they all bad or wrong.

I think this is vital so that we do not make the mistake common to many alternative thinkers of dismissing Western medicine, its research and all its medicines and treatments in a reactionary manner. The issues with it lie not usually in the people within medicine, or much of the science or research behind it, or many of the life-saving, life-improving technologies, nor in the medicines themselves, but the underlying philosophies and unconscious structural tendencies that inform them, and the means of communication that have been historically accepted. If we are unaware of these we can react and respond in a purely emotional manner, without being able to understand the root causes of the problem. Without understanding what is *wrong* with the way things are now, we cannot hope to make things *better*. Our response will be merely reactionary, not truly creative or empowering.

The following is a potted history of patriarchal medicine, just a brief (and most definitely unobjective) overview. Volumes have been written on various aspects of this topic, but many are so academic that only those of us who have studied philosophy, psychology or cultural theory at university, who are privileged to have graduate-level education or access to impressive libraries have been able to avail of them. If this is a topic that you would like to explore further, I point you to the resources section for a plethora of books on the subject far more expert than my own.

SICKNESS AND THE PATRIARCHY

Patriarchy is just a container in which to hide the toxic parts of our human selves. Directly and indirectly, patriarchy is a system of totalitarian control that supports and promotes the conditions – like racism, scapegoating, climate warming and unregulated gun ownership – absolute prerequisites for violence and chaos to erupt. Patriarchy is an umbrella term under which culture, capitalism and its other elements are mere 'shell corporations' of male control. Rather than a means to an end, patriarchy is an end in itself, and the most serious threat to public health that the world has ever known.[38]
Robert Hartman

It is important to remember that the medical system we have today is not a static entity, nor does it define all those who work within it. Indeed, many of the problematic elements of Western medicine that twentieth century philosophers such as Ivan Illich and Michel Foucault, as well as radical feminists including the Boston Women's Health Collective, Barbara Ehrenreich and Deirdre English observed have been addressed, albeit superficially.

The System we have today is very different to the one that they were writing about in the 1970s. And that in turn was very different to the one of the 1950s. So much has changed for the better. A hospital of today is in many ways a far more humane and safe place to be than in 1850, which again was far better than in 1550. Mental health care, though stretched at the seams, is far more advanced than it was in the 1950s, in the days of enforced lobotomies. Elements of consent have certainly been added to care, from careful screening for official medical trials, to the introduction of 'Do Not Resuscitate' forms, birth plans and consent waivers. Progress has been, and is continually being, made, especially in technological terms.

However, it is vital to acknowledge that Western medicine has 'advanced' time and again through non-consenting experiments on tens of thousands of prisoners, mental health patients, Black, Latino and Native peoples, women, and of course millions of animals. From electroshock therapy, to the development of the contraceptive pill tested on poor Puerto Rican women and fatally withholding medical treatment in trials with African American men. Not to mention the vast amounts of medical data gleaned from sadistic Nazi scientists and covert CIA programs, as well as chemicals, medicines and surgical techniques developed in times of war: our war on sickness has been rooted in our war on each other.

Whilst it likes to pass itself off as the height of calm, objective evidence-based rationality, patriarchal 'truth' is often founded on strange superstitions upheld by men in odd uniforms, through fear and power. If this sounds like an outrageous claim, a glance back in (medical) history can easily convince you of that. Foucault in his classic *Madness and Civilization* shares how a commonly used treatment for mental illness (by the most learned doctors of the time) in the eighteenth century (*after* the Scientific Revolution) was soap-based products: the rationale being that they would cleanse and purify the mind. Other physicians' cures for depression in that era included: honey, chimney soot, wood lice, vinegar and powdered lobster claw.[39] Immersions in water were also to be recommended, but only when done "suddenly and unawares… One need have no fear for their lives."[40] And yet the women treated by these strange cures were the ones who were considered crazy by their culture, and their doctors the sane ones to be trusted!

This is history, you cry, things have moved on. In some ways, yes. But these behaviours and treatments form the accepted and acceptable foundations of Western medicine. They too were once considered the scientifically-proven gold-standard in treatment. Because the System said so.

Western medicine is encoded with the philosophical beliefs of patriarchy. The medical establishment is an integral part of the dominant System, charged with the care (and control) of the human bodies and minds of all citizens. And whilst the majority of the individuals that represent the medical system today, male and female, are in the healing professions for all the right reasons, they and we are often blind to the violent bias of the System that shapes medicine.

ANCIENT ROOTS

The roots of the Western medical tradition weave back in history to pre-Christian times, to ancient Greece and Rome. Our current paradigm is firmly anchored in these ancient patriarchal cultures: our understanding of democracy, our architecture, our sciences, our languages, our myths… many of our major sports and entertainments also stem from theirs.

In medicine the traces are apparent everywhere, you don't even need to dig deep to find them. Take the use of the Rod of Asclepius, for example, a staff entwined by a snake. This ancient symbol associated with a Greek god of healing and medicine is still used by over 60% of medical professionals in the US as part of their branding. It is often confused with the caduceus, the double snake entwined staff of the god Hermes, which is used by another significant percentage of medical services to visually define themselves.

It's not just images that link Western medicine back to ancient, pre-Christian roots, but also its language. Over 90% of the language of medicine is rooted in Greek and to a lesser extent Latin:[41] pathology, diagnosis, prognosis, mammogram, mastectomy, cystitis, hygiene, urethra, hysteria, hysterectomy… all words that women are familiar with hearing in relation to their female bodies when they deal with medical doctors, come directly from ancient Greek.

As does the root of the word psyche – which is in common use today in defining the branch of doctors dedicated to the mind: psychiatrists and psychologists. Meaning "animating spirit," from the Latin *psyche* and "the soul, mind, spirit; breath; life; the invisible animating principle or entity which occupies and directs the physical body" from Greek *psykhe*. In both these ancient cultures the concept of psyche, often represented symbolically as a butterfly or moth[42] as well as through the myth of Psyche, was far more complex than our own modern understanding of the mind, incorporating multiple levels of reality – energy, mind, life-force, soul and spirit. Furthermore in ancient Greek culture, *soma* – body – was not yet separate from *psyche*, each were interwoven through all aspects of culture including healing.

The celebrated Asclepius whose Rod we still use symbolically, was one of the god Apollo's sons, sharing with him the title, Paean, meaning 'the Healer'. He represented "the healing aspect of the medical arts; his daughters are Hygieia ('Hygiene', the goddess/personification of health, cleanliness, and sanitation), Iaso (the goddess of recuperation from illness), Aceso (the goddess of the healing process), Aglæa (the goddess of the glow of good health), and Panacea (the goddess of universal remedy)."[43] As we can see from this, the ancient Greek understanding of health and healing was far broader than our Western scientific concerns of curing disease. And those who followed Asclepius used temples as their healing spaces, and incorporated the use of snakes and the importance of dreams as vital tools for healing the mind alongside the body.

The Hippocratic Oath is perhaps the most enduring thing we inherited from the ancient Greeks. Most of us are familiar with the term – but have you actually ever read it? I know I hadn't before writing this book. I think it might surprise you, which is why I share in full the modern version that is still taught in medical schools today, as well as the opening and closing lines of the ancient version.

Modern version of The Hippocratic Oath[44]

I swear to fulfil, to the best of my ability and judgment, this covenant:

I will respect the hard-won scientific gains of those physicians in whose steps I walk, and gladly share such knowledge as is mine with those who are to follow.

I will apply, for the benefit of the sick, all measures which are required, avoiding those twin traps of overtreatment and therapeutic nihilism.

I will remember that there is art to medicine as well as science, and that warmth, sympathy, and understanding may outweigh the surgeon's knife or the chemist's drug.

I will not be ashamed to say 'I know not,' nor will I fail to call in my colleagues when the skills of another are needed for a patient's recovery.

I will respect the privacy of my patients, for their problems are not disclosed to me that the world may know. Most especially must I tread with care in matters of life and death. If it is given me to save a life, all thanks. But it may also be within my power to take a life; this awesome responsibility must be faced with great humbleness and awareness of my own frailty. Above all, I must not play at God.

I will remember that I do not treat a fever chart, a cancerous growth, but a sick human being, whose illness may affect the person's family and economic stability. My responsibility includes these related problems, if I am to care adequately for the sick.

I will prevent disease whenever I can, for prevention is preferable to cure.

I will remember that I remain a member of society, with special obligations to all my fellow human beings, those sound of mind and body as well as the infirm.

If I do not violate this oath, may I enjoy life and art, respected while I live and remembered with affection thereafter. May I always act so as to preserve the finest traditions of my calling and may I long experience the joy of healing those who seek my help.

I think that this oath holds the same vision of healing most of us aspire to, there is nothing evil or greedy or dangerous or insidious in this physicians' professional covenant: prevention is better than a cure, treating a sick person as a person first, and above all not playing God.

But I believe that the beginning and end of the classical vow are even more powerful, and show some of the soul that has been clinically removed from modern medicine. The original Hippocratic Oath began with the invocation "I swear by Apollo the Physician and by Asclepius and by Hygieia and Panacea and by all the gods …" and it finished this way: "If I transgress it and swear falsely, may the opposite of all this be my lot."[45]

So if these are the roots of modern medicine… what went wrong?

CHURCH AS FOUNDATION

The problem is not religion or God. The actual problem is authoritarianism, mixed with the desire to angrily impose one's personal, apparently idealistic, beliefs on others.
Abhijit Naskar

The next step in the development of Western medicine was the one and a half thousand year influence of the Christian church. Regardless of your own personal beliefs or philosophies, the State you inhabit was most likely founded on the philosophy that for a couple of millennia has asserted that man was made in God the Father's image, placed by God to rule on Earth, empowered by God to act as God-like in authority over the Earth's resources, other creatures, and all other peoples – women, children and people of colour.

Christian values and stories, Church-owned lands and institutions, Church-approved teachings have formed the foundation of the dominant European and colonial patriarchal cultures. Religious orders ran – and still run – many hospitals worldwide. In fact, the Catholic Church is the largest non-governmental provider of healthcare services in the world:[46] as of 2010, the Catholic Church's own Pontifical Council stated that the Church manages 26% of the world's healthcare facilities.[47] (Please see the Appendix for my personal reflections on the impact on the Catholic Church on healthcare in Ireland.)

There has always been a compassionate side to most religions. In Christianity it stems directly from the example of Jesus, who dedicated his life to healing and ministering to the poor and sick. In times when most ordinary people were not able to either access or afford medical care, this was a lifeline. But one that tended to come with strings attached: spiritual obligation, obedience and compliance.

Sickness and its care have been closely bound up with religious judgement and morality for most of the past two millennia within European and European-colonial cultures. Goodness has equalled health, health is wealth, and wealth proves success and rewards you for your spiritual goodness. And so the infinite feedback loop of privilege turns. Whereas if you are sick, and poor enough not to be able to afford the healthcare you need, it has been interpreted as a reflection on your morals, a public exposure of your personal failings and hidden crimes or sins: it is a sign that you have angered God and need to atone for this. To be sick is to be contagious, not just physically but morally. To be sick is to be bad or wrong. To be sick is to be pitied or shunned. Being sick, rather than being acknowledged and treated as a vulnerable and integral part of all our humanity, has instead been culturally denied, and often treated politically and morally.

There is a long and dark history of spiritual practices forcibly given alongside and in the name of medicine, attached to the Church's involvement with healthcare. One that many prefer to turn a blind eye to. But when these institutions are the ones that are being exposed for their abuse of vulnerable women and children who were under their care right up to the late twentieth century, when these institutions are still holding undue influence over secular law and medicine, it is vital that we pay attention and demand change. For many, many women, for many, many reasons the involvement of religious bodies in the care of *our* bodies and souls is simply unacceptable: it carries with it an indelible stain of unacknowledged trauma and abuse.

A TANGLED SYSTEM OF CONTROL

As we have begun to see, the Western medical establishment was built within the patriarchal system, and has a long, tangled history with the powers of the State, penal system and Church. Over successive centuries the various tentacles of the State have been interwoven, enforcing the morality and norms of each era through control, containment, punishment and medical treatment.

In more recent times the power of the System has been overseen, corrected and tempered by democracy, that proud Western tradition, developed once again by our ancient Greek and Roman forebears. But for centuries, as Western medicine was developing, democracy had been abandoned by Europeans in favour of absolutist patriarchal rule by kings, dukes, lords and militias. The rule of law was not democratically overseen but a political tool of subjugation and threat. Ditto its organs of control religion and medicine. Only in the past century has the idea of democracy been extended to all citizens, and the concept of consent is still very much a battleground being fought by women and people of colour.

Democracy was not the dominant social model for the majority of the history of Western medicine. This is perhaps illustrated best in the establishment of hospitals, prisons and asylums and the often unseen connections between these places.

The first major hospital was built in Europe in the fifteenth century to contain plague victims after the population of Venice was decimated time and again by the plague brought in by rats carried on their trading ships. They decided to build vast warehouse-like buildings on an uninhabited island to sequester any people who showed symptoms of plague. With no medicines and only the most basic of care, most died there. But Venice's economy and population thrived.[48]

The same was done on a smaller scale with sufferers of leprosy in the Middle Ages all over Europe. Again this hospitalisation was more like involuntary confinement, paid for by Church and State.[49]

When leprosy died out in Europe in the seventeenth century these buildings' purpose was transformed. Now it was the poor and the mad who were confined – again usually against their will – in them. They became the poor houses, containing those who were deemed uncontrollable, dangerous or unsavoury to society.

And on we move, some of these buildings become hospitals, some prisons, some mental asylums. All containing those that society finds unpalatable. Behind high walls and locked gates the shadow side of humanity is kept, the ones that there is no place for in our culture.

The money for the facilities came from those who had done well in the System. Their values and morals shaped the institutions their money built, their ownership of the land that was used gave them power over what was done within the walls. These were places to experiment with new philosophies: some were visionary in positive ways, others cruel and callous.

But the ones treated in these places, were those who had been broken by the very System that now cared for them – through birth or economics, those felled by infection or bad fortune, those who had received a lack of care were contained, controlled, hidden, silenced so that the illusion of the good life could march on unchallenged by all those who disproved or disrupted it.[50] Has much changed?

TRAUMA

I do not want to be here, but nobody else can help me.

This is my last chance.

If I behave myself there will be ice cream.

It is the ice cream that makes me feel better. Not this.

But it seems like nobody ever asks me what I want.

Nobody asks me what I cannot say.

Nobody wants to know what is blocking my throat beyond the pus and the swelling. There is no way of speaking what cannot be spoken.

Everybody needs me to be quiet. To be a Good Girl.

And so I am.

My 'problem' is mapped by the doctor in the white coat, in his words. He defines the area that he specialises in: my ears, nose and throat. My ears, nose and throat are the centre of his universe, for these moments, now. The rest of my body is a black hole, an unexplored universe.

The office is grand, a high ceilinged baroque room with expensive wallpaper. A line of chairs snakes its way down the narrow corridor filled with sick, desperate people. Walking into his office I feel so small, like Alice down the rabbit hole. I sit on the chair opposite him, legs dangling in space.

He arches his fingers like a church steeple, and his eyebrows like a judge. This man is an important doctor, the framed certificates on the wall attest to that. The smart brass plaque on the white wall under the columned entrance. Each letter after his name proof of his mastery and brilliance. Proof of his unassailable authority. *Is he God?* I wonder.

If he is, I do not like God.

I do not trust him. But no one will listen to me. I am only a girl. I am the one who is sick, he is the one with the power to do what others cannot: make me better.

But he does not. Cannot.

He talks about me, over me. I am used to this. I am only the sick one, therefore I do not hold the answers. There is something wrong with me. He will fix it.

Except he hasn't fixed it yet.

But we keep coming back. Knowing somehow that the fault must lie with me.

I lie back on the paper-covered bed.

He leans forward, hands around my throat, fingers squeezing, *palpating* he calls it. It feels like he is choking me. I remember the command: I am silent. I do not like this. But I know it hurts more when I wriggle or scream. I imagine the people who have lain here before me, trying not to scream.

I must not scream.

In my ears I hear the echoes of a hundred thousand silenced screams.

His treatment table is laid out in the centre of the room. Pristine white, this is his altar space, and I the sacrifice.

I cannot see what he is doing, I hear a slapping and washing and a clang of metal.

I am just a little girl. I do not know this now, but when I am a woman, I will still just be a little girl.

He approaches the table with his assistant, both are wearing masks and white rubber gloves, a tray of bright shiny instruments beside him: the torture rack. Which will he use today? The scalpel, the scraper, the thumb racks... What will remain of me? My whole body is shaking now, my breath caught, I want to run. He is the predator and I the prey. But they are two, I am one, they are big and I am small. This room is theirs.

I want to scream, but who will help me? The smell of his gloves and the antiseptic hits the back of my throat. The bright light behind him makes me feel as though this is the inquisition. God himself is coming down from the sky. I escape from my body and watch it lying there from the ceiling.

Open wide... he commands.

My mind knows it must obey. My body cannot. Will not. It is frozen with fear. I use every part of myself to will it to, it opens a tiny crack.

Hands descend to force it further open.

Lie still.

I hear screams.

Shhhh, don't make a fuss, we're not going to hurt you. It's not just me, the room is full of the ghosts of screaming women, silenced. 'Treated'. 'Helped'.

I don't want to be helped. I want to be free.

His head looms further down.

The screams have stopped but hot tears are running down out of eyes that will not open any more.

His fingers are in my mouth.

His fingers are down my throat.

I am gagging and crying and dribbling. I am an animal, wild and crazed. I try to move away but I am pinned by the assistant.

Afterwards there is a shaking of hands, an appointment for next week, a light chat about the weather.

The girl in the room has gone.

Where I do not know.

But her body will be brought back here next week. And the week after.

Open wide,

Don't scream.

Until one day her father brings her. He hears the scream. He hears me.

Stop!

He says, pulling himself to his full height.

He takes me by the hand and we walk out together.

I never go back.

It turns out that there were other doctors after all. Other ways. Doctors who do not stick their fingers down my throat. Doctors with strange machines with big leather headphones that go beep. Doctors who also do not ask me what they do not want to hear. What I cannot say.

Doctors that do not hurt me.

But nor can they cure me.

What struck me most, with all these doctors, is how sure they were.

How sure my parents were.

That somewhere in those books, behind the wire-framed glasses were the answers. That they could see inside me and make me better.

But none of them ever could, ever did. Nobody ever saw me. Not until I was a grown woman, and I saw myself and found someone who could see it too.

Instead I had to go along with each of their far-flung plans – banana flavoured antibiotics, no dairy, foul tasting herbs, each of them handed over as a magical elixir that would fix me.

But they never did.

I learned then, at five or six, a truth that I could not bring myself to speak aloud for another thirty years: that the doctors know far less than we all thought.

Each visit to a hospital as the years progressed and different maladies presented themselves, each proved incurable, inscrutable to the educated gazes of doctors who would prick me and poke me and test me and keep me in for observation and write notes and give drugs. But each time, every time, it was my body that got better by itself.

Each and every time.

But still I wanted to believe. To trust in what I had been taught, what our culture believes: that this medicine will make me better.

DOCTOR/PRIEST

In the secular world of modern medicine we try desperately to rescue ourselves from the grasp of the Unknowable. Doctors have supplanted the gods, deciding when life begins and ends, working miracles, and taking credit for their successes.
Kat Duff, *The Alchemy of Illness*

The Enlightenment [...] with its secular priests presiding over temples of Wisdom, Reason and Nature, [...]the triumph of light over darkness, of sun over moon, of day over night, of reason, tolerance and love over passion.
Isaac Kramnick, *The Portable Enlightenment Reader*

The next major influence on the evolution of Western medicine was the Enlightenment, a philosophical and scientific movement of the seventeenth and eighteenth centuries led by thinkers including

Réné Descartes ("I think, therefore I am"), Isaac Newton (father of Newtonian physics), Francis Bacon (father of the scientific method), Adam Smith (father of free-market capitalism and the invisible hand), Benjamin Franklin (founding father of the modern US constitution). These men indelibly shaped our modern era, replacing the enforced beliefs of the Church and the cruelty of the 'dark ages', with the 'light' of logic and rationality. At the very heart of the Enlightenment project was the desire to understand all existence with the power of the mind. Scepticism (a philosophical approach rooted in the tenets of an ancient Greek cult) became the new watchword for this movement, replacing the superstitious beliefs of times gone by. And so doubt replaced faith as the guiding light of our culture.

It is hardly surprising then that the cultural void left by the diminishment of religion was quickly filled by the honouring of science. The vaunted role of priest was taken by the scientist, the "natural philosopher king". One patriarchal system seamlessly replaced another using a very similar framework.

In the Western world, the role of both doctor and priest have been almost exclusively held by men until very, very recent times: just as only men were allowed to be direct channels of the Authorized God's word as official priests, only men were trusted to be effective scientists and medical practitioners. Where once the eldest son of a family would have become a priest to gain respect for his family, prestige and a viable income, now he became a doctor.

Science is still a male-dominated field, even today (note the preponderance of Women in STEM programs in recent years, and the attempts to entice more girls to study science). And scientists have retained an unquestionable authority as those who most understand the workings of the universe, whose opinions are most respected. It is to them we still confer the power to understand and manage life and death, and to hand down accepted truths, in the way that priests of old previously did. In both these fields it was the male intercessor who had the connection to divine knowledge and therefore power. Not the individual in need of healing. Certainly not if she were female. Or poor. Or of colour.

And so only the white male soul, body and mind came to define the norm, against which all others were categorized, judged, measured, and so often found lacking, silenced and pushed into the shadows.

Where once the Church would have stepped in to save us, now the medical establishment does. The hospital has become our new place of worship, with doctors our new saviours.

And many, many of us have been deeply traumatised in the process.

A LOSS OF SOUL

The relationship to the world that modern science fostered and shaped now appears to have exhausted its potential. It is increasingly clear that the relationship is missing something. It fails to connect with the most intrinsic nature of reality, and with natural human experience. It is now more of a source of disintegration and doubt than a source of integration and meaning. It produces what amounts to a state of schizophrenia, completely alienating man as an observer from himself as a being. Classical modern science described only the surface of things, a single dimension of reality. And the more dogmatically science treated it as the only dimension, as the very essence of reality, the more misleading it became.
Vaclav Havel, former Czech President,
The Art of the Impossible

Most cultures have an understanding of humans as being more than simply their physical bodies. Each has their own native knowledge of the existence of one or more energetic bodies connected to a greater spirit or soul. This essential part of our beings, the soul, is understood to transcend the body's physical limitations, travel in dreams, in prayer, in ceremony and beyond death, becoming disconnected or confused during trauma. The individual soul is understood to have direct connections with its host body, as well as with other spirits and souls in both this world and non-material realms, alongside larger universal forces and qualities such as fate, healing, love, death and the divine. This is the self that feels connection to people, animals and places, the part of us that motivates our passionate action. This part cannot be observed directly but illuminates our bodies during our lifetimes, holds the essence of what we are and continues after our death.

It seems only in the self-proclaimed most advanced civilization in history that this core part of humanity is dismissed: ironically it seems that the greatest lesson of the Enlightenment project was to be sceptical of the existence and meaning of our very selves. Under modern Western science and philosophy, the body became only what we could see and touch: an object, subject to intensive scrutiny and observation.

In modern medicine the *being* part of humanity is still widely ignored, whilst our material bodies, which were once considered under Christian thought as simply vessels of clay for our immortal souls, have morphed into our main reality: the Enlightenment vision of "man as machine"[51] has been almost completely realized.

The surgical doctor of the Industrial Age was promoted to doing the *real* 'work' of repairing the body and its mechanics, with mind doctors coming later to deal with the pesky, nebulous realm of mental illness, which due to their intangibility were deemed less 'real'. Priests were relegated to the least visible, and therefore least real: the soul and spiritual connection and to some extent the wellbeing of the human community. For the first time in humanity the human body was philosophically and psychologically distanced from the mind, and both detached from the soul.

Today our doctors and hospitals still minister to the physical wounds, to the bodily condition, as though the whole person can be detached from the illness. We nod our heads to the notion of soul – there is a chapel in most hospitals, and priests are called on to give last rites – but there is no location on any medical diagram for the soul. Mind and consciousness are generally understood as merely energetic emanations of the brain. We do surgery on bodies in much the same way that we fix our cars. We give medication in the same way that we kill weeds in our fields with herbicides. The body and mind, where they can be tested and acted upon, are treated separately. The soul which inhabits that body, the "ghost in the machine",[52] has become secondary to these: an easily overlooked afterthought. As a culture we have learned to dismiss and ignore that which we cannot understand with our minds.

There is, in most cultures, an acknowledgement of the mysterious nature of sickness and healing, and a belief that the gods, spirits or ancestors hold some sway over the unknowable forces that govern life and death. And still today most of us, even if we do not consider ourselves religious, pray in some manner for the healing of loved ones who are sick. Even today we speak of 'miraculous' cures that have confounded the medical profession. We still have a deep-rooted, some may say irrational, belief that healing is mysterious and that it goes beyond what is simply done to the body by the hands of men, despite all we have learned in school.

In most traditional societies the role of healer or medicine person (which could be held by a man or a woman) combined the guidance and healing of both bodymind and soul, as the two were seen as indivisible: both were vital for life and health. The health of the individual was seen within the context of both the human community, ancestors and spirits, and the natural world. Illness was the sign that something was out of balance in one or more of these realms. Ritual, ceremony and spiritual expression were seen as a vital part of navigating the realm of illness and coming back to health.

We have lost this in our culture. Sickness has become meaningless, just as human life and culture have become soulless. Western medicine has focused far more on the individual organs and their functioning in isolation, rather than looking at the whole bio-energetic system and the relationships between all its parts. Just as in our culture we place all our attention on the individual, not the healthy functioning of the system of relationships in which the individual is embedded.

Life has been divided against itself again and again as a direct result of our philosophical and scientific approach. Our culture has created intellectual and emotional schisms: between body and mind, human and nature, between 'primitive' and 'advanced' human cultures, between masculine and feminine, East and West, between arts and sciences, home and world, and ultimately between life and death. Like splitting the atom, the potential for disaster is high.

The connections that were severed in the Enlightenment re-wrote our understanding of ourselves. For the first time in our existence, what it meant to be human was reduced from being an integral expression of the divine, the natural world, the race, community and family, to solely being contained within the boundaries of the physical body, controlled by the individual brain and genetic code. And whilst this surgical removal of the beingness of humanity enabled many philosophical and technological advances that had previously been prohibited due to moral or religious concerns, it has come at a high price: our human wellness.

THE MEDICALISATION OF BODY AND MIND

The medicalisation of women's bodies is the biggest land-grab on the planet.
Dr Marion Gluck, *Femme: Women Healing the World*

The actual preoccupation of psychiatry is nothing less than the quasi-academic compartmentalization of certain states of experience into formally reduced types of 'illness' that are then logically disposable in the field of curing.
David Cooper, introduction to Foucault's *Madness and Civilization*

After European colonialists had finished exploring, mapping and colonising the globe by the early nineteenth century, they turned again with renewed vigour to do the same to the human body and mind: the last uncharted territories. In the past century the body and mind have been completely colonised by medical science.

In recent years birth, death, grief, depression, sadness, hyperactivity have all become bonafide 'conditions', to be managed by experts. The idea of them being an integral part of our human journey and experience, each an important rite of passage, each perfectly natural given its circumstances has been lost. Instead they are treated as anomalies, as illnesses to be cured, battles to be won, in order to return the individual to a culturally acceptable and narrow version of 'normal'.

Ivan Illich drew attention to the rampant medicalisation of the body and mind in the 1970s, but since then it has increased, not decreased. Medicalisation refers to the transformation of ordinary human feelings, experiences and life events into 'disorders' that can and 'should' be presided over, defined, diagnosed and treated by doctors, with medication or in a medical setting.

We can see just how fast this process of medicalisation has been in the young field of psychiatry. In 1952, the first edition of the Diagnostic and Statistical Manual (DSM) – the US manual used to diagnose mental health conditions – outlined 106 categories of mental pathology. Including homosexuality as a psychiatric illness established the book's dubious credentials for medicalising innate human traits. The third edition, DSM-III, published in 1980, less than thirty years later, contained over twice the number of official disorders, a whopping 265.[53] Where did they all come from... and why?

As a society, it seems, we have marched headlong into the habit of searching for active medicine to cure the surface symptoms of our suffering, searching anxiously for treatments and specialists outside ourselves. As our physical and mental discomfort have increased, we have become more and more desperate to find someone or something to make us better. With medical knowledge, technology and products so readily accessible, we automatically jump straight into looking for medical solutions to issues which may only be partly medical problems. Once we are set on looking for a 'solution', the illness is then locked in as the 'problem'[54] to be gotten rid of, whatever the cost.

Along with medicalisation comes the belief that the 'problem' lies with the individual, and that sickness is any deviation outside of a very narrowly defined 'norm'. What is normal is being constantly reduced, and the human complexity of the individual tends to be lost amongst labels and symptoms. Meanwhile those in other branches of the System demand official labels in order to deviate from their new standardized norms and act with compassion or offer support.

This was being recognised by the US government as a major issue back in the 1970s, when a Senate subcommittee on health declared, "The problem of dehumanization in healthcare is of increasing concern."[55] As Allan Horwitz and Jerome Wakefield argue in their book, *The Loss of Sadness*, "A mental illness [became] something detectable by observation and classification...in scrapping the possibility that a mental syndrome might be an understandable and proportionate response to a set of external circumstances, psychiatry lost the capacity to identify problems in the fabric of society or economy."[56]

Whilst more of human mental suffering has certainly been more accurately diagnosed and effectively treated using this approach, it is also highly problematic. Society's ills have become our own private illnesses when they are expressed through our individual bodyminds and are then seen as being in need of medication to make them better. Whole swathes of human experience have become pathologised and variations of human brain and body functioning have been medicalised, and therefore medicated, in order to manage and control them.

A NEW GOD: THE RISE AND RISE OF TECHNOLOGY

Medicine is an unacknowledged religion complete with its own language, costumes, and places of worship.
Dr Nicolas Gonzales

Advances in medical technology have risen exponentially in the past century, alongside the medicalisation of the body. Many of them have increased life expectancy and survival rates, from incubators keeping pre-term babies alive, to open heart and brain surgery, stents and pacemakers, chemo and radiotherapy for cancer, sophisticated blood sugar monitoring and external pancreases for diabetes, MRI scanners and ultrasound for a range of diagnostics. Our hi-tech instruments and approaches are the result of hundreds of thousands of doctors' and scientific researchers' dedication. We have come a long way in diagnosis, thanks to these new technologies. We are living longer, more active lives because of them. We are better informed, more connected and empowered by so many aspects of technology. It is a man-made miracle that has the power to transform human suffering.

But also it seems to be serving to further divide us from ourselves. We can see the industrialisation of life, the impinging of expensive and intrusive technology all around us, in every field. Within medicine we see it in the rise of the expensive consultant who is wined and dined by drug companies; the exorbitantly priced pharmaceutical drug that there is no motivation to wean you from; the bombardment (most prominently in the US) of advertising for branded medications; the prescription drug that requires another three to off-set its side effects; the rise and rise in the cost of medical insurance that dictates which treatments are and are not valid or valued.

With these technological advances has come an ever-greater pressure on our doctors and nurses to be godlike too. Within this paradigm, the ordinary person, the patient, is relegated to having to believe and put their faith in the integrity of the charismatic scientist or doctor and their technologies, to accept their authority, methods and motivation without question in order to be 'saved' by them.

Some physicians take their own deification rather literally, as in recent examples of a doctor branding his initials on liver transplants. Or the Irish doctor who spent a career removing women's reproductive organs without consent because of his personal judgements on their sexual and family choices.

For most though, the pressure to be omniscient, and liable to be litigated against when one fails is a high price indeed. It tends to make medical professionals wary of honest interactions with patients, more likely to rely on technology rather than their own senses, more likely to make – and cover up – mistakes due to technological errors.

The current medical system simply does not allow for the full humanity of either patient or doctor. And the mental illness brought on by stress and anxiety is not just occurring in patients, it is running at its highest level ever amongst doctors and nurses too.[57]

Western medicine is on life support.

MEDICINE QUESTIONS

Do you experience medical treatment/personnel/institutions as patriarchal – in what ways?

How has gender impacted:

- *Medical issues you have?*

- *Doctors' attitudes to your pain or suffering?*

- *Doctors' treatment of you as a person?*

How has religion impacted:

- *Medical issues you have?*

- *Doctors' attitudes to your pain or suffering?*

- *Doctors' treatment of you as a person?*

Do you see any connections between medicine and religion?

What happens if you disagree with a doctor?

Have you ever felt shamed in treatment? Have you ever been traumatised?

THE DEATH OF CARE

SICKNESS
– THE LAST GROWTH INDUSTRY IN PATRIARCHY

The spirit of this agenda originates with the Enlightenment. But those who have exploited it best are those with an interest in social control, very often for private profit.
William Davies, *The Happiness Industry: How the Government and Big Business Sold Us Wellbeing*

What is strange is that despite advances in medicine and technology, despite our comparative prosperity, peace and easy lives here in the modern West, every year more and more of us are becoming permanent residents, rather than occasional visitors, of what Susan Sontag referred to as "the kingdom of the sick".[58]

In 2012, 117 million Americans (almost half the population) were living with chronic illness. One in four adults had two or more chronic health conditions,[59] accounting for nearly 75% of all health-care spending.[60] In the UK doctors write 1 billion prescriptions via the National Health Service (NHS). Every year.[61] For a population of 65 million.[62] This number is even more staggering when you take into consideration the fact that it represents a rise of almost two thirds compared to just a decade ago. In the US the number is just shy of 3 billion prescriptions,[63] with 48.7% of the population using at least one prescription drug each month. We are leaning heavily on the prescription pad to try to make us better.

In the UK 90% of these prescriptions were given free. But the NHS is faltering at the edge of collapse after years of government under-investment and ever-growing demands on its resources. In the US prescription drugs are so expensive that some states are shipping in cheaper alternatives from Canada.[64] Chemotherapy for breast cancer that in the UK costs the NHS just £4,500 per patient is charged at £105,000 per patient in the US.[65] Personal healthcare costs have most than doubled in less than fifteen years in America. Whilst between 2004 and 2014, the percentage of the US population under sixty-five with private health insurance obtained through the workplace declined almost 10%.[66] For millions the healthcare they need lies out of reach. Healthcare reforms are a political hot potato, thrown backwards and forwards between Democrats and Republicans. And still chronic illness keeps growing. Especially amongst women.

With the ability to save lives has always come power, prestige, influence and in capitalist times, money. The medicalisation of the body and its illnesses in patriarchal culture has directly led to their commodification. It could be argued that our culture is profiting richly from our suffering.

This raises some uncomfortable questions, such as: Who does it benefit when we are sick? What if the way that our culture is set up and maintained is making us sick? What if what is really making us sick is not being researched – but rather the research is going to where the money is and the kudos is, not where more complex but potentially unprofitable answers and medicines lie? What if our being sick is of benefit to our culture – keeping us powerless, indebted and adding copiously to the GDP? Typing that last bit gave me chills down my spine. And not the good kind. It sounds like a hideous dystopia or a wild conspiracy theory. But it's a possibility. Look at our economic system and you see that a cancer patient, a long-term medicated patient of low earning capacity is worth more to the economy than a well person, what with doctors' pay and hospital charges, medications, health insurance... Is the System invested in creating, discovering and treating our sickness, rather than promoting our health?

THE MAGIC BULLET

Within the voiced pain of a woman lies the power to bring the world
As we know it,
This bright, shiny, hard world,
To its knees.

The majority of people in the Western world are now drugged just to allow them to survive this culture: doctors, lawyers, actors, mothers, presidents, cleaners, emergency responders, models, athletes, terrorists, shop workers, students, administrators… and me. We are drugged to cope with late nights, early mornings, endless stress, too much work, not enough time, too few resources, rushed meals, pressure, pressure, pressure. So we swallow down our drug(s) of choice: the antacids, the paracetamol, we hide the vodka bottles, take sleeping pills, pop a Xanax, Fentanyl, drink coffee to energise, sugar to give us energy, take antidepressants to numb the darkness, perhaps a snort of coke so we can keep going a bit longer, a drag on a joint to relax us, brain stimulants to keep us alert and yet more painkillers to numb the sensation of living.

Medication takes many forms. Some keeps us alive. Some kills us slowly. Some makes life worth living and some makes its own problems which in turn need yet more medication. Some numbs pain, eases blood flow, fights bacteria, turns down the volume on our anxiety, reduces swelling, helps us sleep, eases constipation. It helps our bodies to do what they are currently unable to do themselves. As a temporary crutch whilst we put in place the other supports that are needed, it can be a lifesaver: a bridge back to health. And if no other supports exist for a condition, it is a permanent lifesaver. Medication is necessary at many times, for many conditions. It is often a vital piece of the puzzle.

I know this from personal experience.

Over the course of writing this book I found myself in the midst of a breakdown, attempting to manage my children's medical conditions and finally caved to taking a tranquilising medication. For a few days. On my terms. In tiny doses. Because life was so far outside of my control. My system was so exhausted. And in order to make it through the System for my family, that was what I needed. After resisting for years and years, after failed medication attempts before, I knew that whilst we got all our other supports and approaches in place, I needed something to keep me functioning.

I was very resistant to the idea of taking it. And I am very, very grateful for it.

But it wasn't enough. And antidepressants took their place and became what made me able to function in the midst of the chaos.

And I am very grateful for them too. Just like I am very grateful for paracetamol when I have a migraine. But they are not the answer, not a long-term solution. They are a stop gap. A numbing, whilst I can find a way to heal the root cause. A way to keep the show on the road.

But this is not how medication is used by the majority of the medical profession. Pharmaceuticals are seen as the answer. Stop the pain. Job done. Next.

The prescription of antidepressants to 34.4 million Americans in 2013-2014 [was] up from 13.4 million just 15 years earlier. And this pervasive prescribing continues despite the lack of proof of the drugs' long-term effectiveness; their mixed results even with short-term treatment; the frequent side-effects — weight gain, gastrointestinal problems and sexual dysfunction — that are themselves depressing. Meanwhile, we are paying the prohibitive financial costs of depression — an estimated annual average of $210.5bn in treatment and lost productivity.[67]

Pharmaceutical medication is not the one-size-fits-all answer for most sicknesses that our culture treats it as. It may address some symptoms but not the bigger picture of why we are sick in the first place, nor how we can stay well in the future.

And there is another problem, if you're a woman: the majority of medication is and has historically been administered by men, formulated by men, funded by men, tested on men. Even when the majority recipients are female. According to Dr Paula Johnson, director of Women's Health at Brigham and Women's Hospital, "Women are still not included in clinical research in numbers that reflect the prevalence and impact of disease in women… The science that informs medicine – including the prevention, diagnosis, and treatment of disease – routinely fails to consider the crucial impact of sex and gender."[68]

In the cutting words of Alyson McGregor's rousing TED talk "Why medicine often has dangerous side effects for women": "A recent Government accountability study revealed that 80% of the drugs withdrawn from the market are due to side effects on women... It turns out that those cells used in that laboratory, they're male cells, and the animals used in the animal studies were male animals, and the clinical trials have been performed almost exclusively on men."[69]

And there is another issue, whatever your age or gender: medication also tends to cause a whole raft more symptoms that in turn need medicating. And so the wheels of big pharma keep turning, alleviating not only the initial illnesses but all their side effects.

Medication has become the only way for the majority of humans to survive the internal and external pain that is our daily reality. And we're all medicating more and more just to keep up with the Joneses. We're all trying to keep the mask on, stop it from slipping, stop our minds and bodies from rebelling. We're being extra careful not to let our crazy hang out, not to reveal the rashes and scars that we bear. We're holding it all in, just, thanks to medication.

It seems that it doesn't matter what we suffer in private. As long as it stays private. As long as we don't appear sick to others. As long as we don't seem contagious. As long as we're not branded sick.

Because sick sticks.

It changes the way people treat us. Changes the box they put us into. We become creatures of pity or avoidance or charity. We become difficult, untrustworthy, needy, weak and unreliable.

And we just want an easy life. And we need to keep our job to pay the bills and keep a roof over our heads. And who else could look after the kids?

So we learn how to keep up appearances, keep it in, unaware that almost everyone else is doing the same in private, some more, some less, but we're all putting the cream on our rashes, taking the tablets, seeing the therapist, avoiding dairy or crowded places. Popping pill after pill. Just one more drink. Hiding our realities from others, too scared of judgement. Pretending to be someone else. Okay. Happy. Nothing to see here.

And why wouldn't we? We have a fundamental human need to belong. We are tribal creatures. To belong is to be protected, to stay safe.

And to do this we believe we have to be well, so that we don't get abandoned or shunned.

And so we're reaching for the quick fix, for short term solutions to chronic problems. Hoping that they will fix the problem again. And again. And again. But in this short-termism we're allowing ourselves to take our eyes off a need for long-term solutions, which are far more subtle and complex. And we're handily overlooking the impact of these stop-gap solutions on the individuals taking them, let alone their communities and the environment.

And we keep on focusing on the individual.

But it's not just the occasional individual who has a problem now.

The medication is enabling our communal denial and the only ones who can't live in denial are the ones the medication doesn't work for. Or who can't get any.

But it seems like we're too overwhelmed and exhausted to care.

THE DEATH OF CARE

Positive thinking has made itself useful as an apology for the crueller aspects of the market economy... The flip side of positivity is thus a harsh insistence on personal responsibility: if your business fails or your job is eliminated, it must be because you didn't try hard enough, didn't believe firmly enough in the inevitability of your success.
Barbara Ehrenreich, *Smile or Die: How Positive Thinking Fooled America and The World*

The magic bullet has missed and has killed care.
We don't have time to care anymore.
We don't have the energy left to care.
We are replacing care with chemicals.

A close relative is in hospital as I write, transferred from another for emergency surgery, she spent the night on a trolley in the corridor. This was despite having extensive private medical insurance. She was given a sleeping pill, to help her rest. And this hit home hard for me. It is cheaper, easier, far more efficient to knock people out – to medicate them – than provide what they need: a quiet room to rest, nurses on call. One simple, cheap pill means you can cut corners everywhere else. A medicated patient is less trouble. Care costs, chemicals are cheaper. So chemicals win.

In many ways and places technology itself is becoming a new god, supplanting the human skills of listening and caring: the computer replacing the empathy of a smile, a nod, the clouding of eyes with empathetic tears, the cold metal of a machine replacing the warmth of human hands on skin and the unquantifiable healing that they can bring. In the words of a former editor of the *Journal of the American Medical Association*, "I suspect that some atrophy of our diagnostic senses occurred when subjective observation was replaced by objective laboratory data."[70]

We have begun, in many places, to see humans as dispensable. In Japan care assistants are being replaced with robots. Face-to-face doctor appointments are being replaced with on-screen interactions. Phones are being answered by machines whilst office hours are being cut back. In an odd human logic, budget cuts mean that human beings are being replaced by efficient, though expensive, technology. The tender human patient is having to bend herself to the needs and quotas of an unfeeling System.

Each visit to a hospital reminds me of this. Seeing the overworked doctors and nurses huddled round their work stations on computers and phones, filling in forms and flicking through files, whilst the ward is full of sick people, lying passive and helpless in their beds, surrounded by flashing, beeping machines, patiently waiting for their turn, dying for care. They are a seeming afterthought to the bureaucratic engine.

A 2018 study of 20,000 US doctors confirms this, with 71% of physicians saying that they spent over ten hours a week on paperwork and administrative tasks.[71] A figure that has increased year on year. These are hours that are taken away from caring for people, and instead maintaining the medical behemoth.

And so we do away with the expensive counsellors, the extra treatment rooms, the nurses, the rehabilitation, the patient garden, the art therapy class, the healthy meals – the tangible, human facets of care, and replace them with pills and machines. When all you're looking at is

the balance sheet, it makes perfect sense. This is what they call rationalisation. This is what happens when numbers and bureaucrats rule:
caring is doled out in pill trays and calculated in spreadsheets.

But this numbing doesn't come cheap to us, the patient healthcare
consumers. We are paying, and paying deeply, for the pain we cannot
bear to feel, the pain we cannot help others deal with, the pain we cannot cure. And we are paying not just with our purses, but with our lives.

We have a serious cultural problem, but rather than work to fix it,
rather than deal with the pain it is causing, we are forcing people to
inhabit it drugged.

PAIN/KILLING

*The risk is that science ends up blaming – and medicating – in-
dividuals for their own misery, and ignores the context that has
contributed to it.*
**William Davies, *The Happiness Industry: How the Government
and Big Business Sold Us Wellbeing***

*Q: Are some treatments just being ignored because they can't be com-
modified by pharma companies?*

*A: Yes, I heard this over and over again from the researchers I in-
terviewed. The majority of clinical trials are funded by pharma
companies, which contributes to a medical system that prioritises the
prescription of drugs, even for conditions such as pain that are strongly
influenced by social and psychological factors. This serves commercial
interests but doesn't necessarily lead to the best outcomes for patients.*[72]
Jo Marchand, author of *Cure*, in a Guardian interview

We are addicted to the magic trick of conjuring away pain.

We have been silencing pain for generations. The pain of wars,
massacres, abuses, immigrations, famines, illness, childbirth... We
are individually, collectively trying to hush the waves of darkness that
keep crashing and crashing belatedly on the shores of our bodyminds.
Trying to keep it down, keep it in, get back to normal. The drugs
may work for a week or a month, but the waves breach their barrier

and we increase our dose. Keep the waters back, the feelings down, the tears in. Nobody wants to hear it, nobody wants to see it. We just don't have the time. We don't have the energy. There is nowhere safe to collapse. We must carry on. And on. And on.

Patriarchal medicine entered into a war on pain and the terms were clear: either we kill it, or it kills us. And they believed that they were winning the war, that we could eradicate pain forever.

But our cultural reliance on magic bullets is backfiring. Rather than eliminating our pain, these bullets are taking our lives. What seemed like the easy option, of opiate painkillers to treat people with back problems, after car accidents and surgery has started an epidemic of opioid addiction. Instead of being the magic answer painkillers have morphed into the most dangerous public health epidemic of the modern age. We are seeing how false the cultural barrier between legal and illegal drugs is.

We see a strange double standard: running a ruthless war on 'illegal' drugs at the same time that more humans than ever in the history of the planet are reliant on psychotropic medicines prescribed by doctors, many of which are of questionable efficacy. And yet some of the so-called illegal drugs (such as MDMA, LSD and marijuana), which are known to be of use in therapeutic settings where there are few effective treatments available, are banned. We have a deep cultural distrust of changing consciousness – and yet every day millions of people have their consciousness legally altered with general anaesthetics and opioid painkillers like codeine and morphine, with alcohol and even with screens. We are against people choosing to use mind-altering substances for personal use, to change their experience of reality, to heal, but are all too happy to prescribe them to ensure people remain functional in this dysfunctional reality when it suits us.

According to the most recent National Survey of Drug Use and Health, just shy of 100 million Americans used, or misused, prescription pain pills in 2015.[73] That's almost 30% of the entire population, with 80% getting hooked on (supposedly non-addictive) opioids after being prescribed them. Described by the US National Institute on Drug Abuse as "a serious national crisis", opioid addictions cost US communities 100 lives a day and $78.5 billion a year.[74]

This escalation in use is not inevitable. Nor is it bad luck. Government, pharmaceutical companies and doctors are complicit in it. According to a special report by The Guardian newspaper, "Pharmaceutical companies spend far more than any other industry to influence politicians. Drugmakers have poured close to $2.5bn into lobbying and funding members of Congress over the past decade."[75] A former head of the Drug Enforcement Agency told the Washington Post. "The drug industry, the manufacturers, wholesalers, distributors and chain drugstores, have an influence over Congress that has never been seen before."[76]

It is no coincidence either that the type of medication that people are becoming addicted to – opioids – "bind to the areas of the brain that control pain and emotions, driving up the levels of the feel-good hormone dopamine."[77] They are drugs that kill not only the physical pain that people are suffering, but also the harrowing emotional pain of living in a dying culture. And we are all ingesting these medications, whether or not we are prescribed them, as most urban water and sea-food is now laced with excreted traces of opioids, antidepressants and the contraceptive pill.[78]

We feel so much pain. Inside, outside. And our culture is not good at dealing with pain. It likes to bury it, numb it, hide it, ignore it. It likes having the ability to carry pain away on one simple pill and have to think no more about it. It prefers to leave aside the messiness of where it came from and why, where it's leading to and how.

Like a thousand fire alarms going off through the night, pain wails as we run in this direction and that, trying to put out the fires. We have been running so long, through the chaos, the smoke, the over-whelm and the adrenaline, our nervous systems are exhausted. But still the alarms are ringing. We long for an end to the suffering. We watch the clock, creeping forwards, each second, each minute and still the pain remains… we look ahead to endless deserts barren of joy, popu-lated only by pain. When will it end? It feels like it will outlast us. We sacrifice more and more of our body, our life, to assuaging the pain, to keeping it at bay. We grow desperate and agitated in the face of its permanence, our concentration, mobility, sociability, identities gradu-ally erased by the pain, until we are living in an invisible circle – just us… and the pain… and its cousins, misery, despair and exhaustion. We lose ourselves to it. Powerless in its grasp.

In our culture we try to separate out physical pain from emotional pain and declare them to be two separate territories. Each of us has a different pain we carry, in different places in our bodies and souls. We have so much pain that we can no longer bear to feel it. We feel so much pain that we are too scared or ashamed to name it. In the abyss we find it hard to know what is my pain, what is your pain, what is our collective pain, what is old pain and what is new, and what can be done about any of it.

We can't take it anymore. It all just hurts.

We are done with it.

And so we swallow down what they offer, hoping to find relief, at last.

CHEMICAL CONSCIOUSNESS

I look at this tiny pill. Will I, won't I?

I will not know its power,

I will not know what I have to lose

Until I swallow it.

I will only know what was mine when it has been taken.

Be a good girl, now.

Trust us.

Open wide.

Close your eyes.

Take a deep breath.

There's nothing to worry about.

I swallow it down.

And wait…

An artificial chemical consciousness takes over.

No anxiety, no fear, no joy, nothing… just blank slowed down awareness. Numbness. White sleep. This is a zombie space that feels as though my soul has been detached from my body and smuggled away somewhere.

I am drifting, but not between the worlds, as I do by myself, in my creative and spiritual practices, but instead into blankness. It is an odd feeling, there are no words or images here, no other worlds, no energy. Just blank nothingness. This is the chemical mind, the man-made medicine-mind.

I don't like it.

I feel my life-force being taken from me, as though it is being sucked against my will down the plughole. There is nothing I can do.

My body remains anxious, my brain is deathly calm, slow motion, dozing off in the middle of the afternoon. I am totally numb, except for mild annoyance at the distraction of what is going on around me: my children. I am in my own world... except it is not my own, it is not my headspace. It is as though someone has crept in and painted everything white. I fight to keep my eyelids open against this warm haze of nothingness.

I drift untethered, my thoughts reach no completion but dangle in mid-air, finding no connection. They seem pointless. Everything seems pointless. Much easier to drift, to stop trying... trying to stand up, trying to concentrate on the words coming towards me from my children's mouths. Is this how a large percentage of the population function: in a desensitised bubble? I don't feel angry or sad, just insulated from the reality going on around me. I have heard people call it a chemical holiday, and that's what it is. It is the pause button I've often longed for... except I'm not in control until it wears off.

In theory I should relax and enjoy this numb drifting feeling, but instead it makes me truly treasure my ordinary consciousness – my feelings, my thoughts, my reality, my creativity like nothing ever has before.

There is a violence in this. A subtle violence. I hesitate to use the word rape. But it is a hijacking of consciousness. A masculine hijacking of my Feminine darkness. Asked for. Taken of my own free will.

Deeply regretted.

I cannot turn it off, only wait it out... and so to sleep again, to the enforced hibernation of my chemically clouded consciousness.

Out of the dull whiteness, bats begin to circle around my head, I cannot stop my eyes from following them. The scream is rising but my body is frozen. Heart pounding. Eyes racing.

Where am I?
Help me! Help me!
Get me out of here,
Bring me home.

MEDICINE QUESTIONS

What has the price of sickness been for you?

What has your experience of the Kingdom of the Sick been?

Medication

Much research in the 1970s and 1980s pointed to the increased efficacy of medical treatments when accompanied by visualisation – the patient visualising the part of the body being treated and what effect the medication or surgical treatment was having on it.[79]

Have you ever used visualisation alongside or instead of medication?

What role have painkillers played in your life until now? How often do you use them? Why do you use them? What other ways do you kill pain?

Can you create an image of pain to represent what it looks or feels like to you? What role does a painkiller play in this?

What role do medications currently play in your healthcare?

Are you grateful for medication, resentful of it, ambivalent about it? Is it a life-saver, a toxic drug, a magic bullet? How has your relationship with it changed over time? How has your dosage changed over time? How much control do you have over your medication regime? Do you understand how it works, and what is in it?

Which of your bodymind systems does your current medication impact and how?

Are you wanting to find a better medication or come off it? What support or information do you need to do so?

Are you aware of any alternative medicines or shifts in dosage that might be gentler on your body?

HEALING ARTS

Pain

Have you ever taken time to examine your pain more closely? What does your pain look like? What colour is it? How big is it? Can you feel it shifting form?

Can you create an image of what pain is for you using colour, texture and different mark making techniques? Does this have any impact on your understanding of pain, or on the pain itself?

MAD, BAD, SAD

◯

A WOMAN'S PLACE

A thousand years ago they would have stoned me for my beliefs.

Five hundred years ago they would have burned me at the stake for witchcraft and heresy.

Two hundred years ago they would have taken my children and locked me in a mental institution for being unstable, for "masturbation, menstrual derangement, depression, political excitement, novel reading, laziness, dissipation of nerves."[80]

A hundred and thirty years ago as a middle-class European woman I would have been forced to my bed, administered opium, smelling salts and cold baths.

Ninety years ago the Americans may have tried to sterilise me because of my genetic lineage.

Eighty years ago the Nazis would have done the same. Or perhaps just killed me outright for my mental and genetic weakness.

Fifty years ago I would have given birth drugged, been tied down, had my baby taken and lived a sedated life – electroshocked against my will.

Today I take antidepressants and anti-anxiety medication and see a therapist – but it is freely chosen and carefully considered. I am free to be me: I mother, write books, make spirals, create online communities, build a woman-based business and am sought out as a speaker.

But today in Ireland I could still be sectioned, if my crazy ever tipped over the edge.

Today under ISIS I would be killed for my views on women and my writings.

Under the Chinese I would be imprisoned as a dissident.

Tomorrow, who knows? The world is changing so fast. And my bodymind knows this.

What others might call anxiety, or paranoid thoughts, I would consider an awareness of history and how women like me – sick women, creative women, political women, mothers, outspoken women, women with mental health issues – have been treated by the patriarchy.

I have a diagnosis that I am public about. I have controversial books with my name on. Things I have chosen of my own free will. Sometimes I am scared that I am digging my own grave, writing my execution or incarceration papers in my own hand.

There but for the grace of tomorrow's System go I.

I live with this knowing every day. That the more of my 'defectiveness' and truth I reveal to the world, the more of myself I expose to the light, the more evidence I give to the System that could decide my fate in the future, that could be used to take my life or liberty.

There has always been a fine line between insanity and insurrection, between the celebrated, outspoken artist and the political dissident or dangerous extremist. It depends on your place in the System. There is the narrowest of gaps between those who deserve our care, and those who need 'taking care of' when times get tough. Sickness, poverty, madness, craziness, criminality, addiction… these have always been interconnected states of being. The main factor in their treatment is the money in your pocket, your family of origin and the allies you have picked up along the way. Some of us get to choose homeopathy, psychotherapy and herbs, others only have the cheap and immediate option of alcohol or painkillers or legal highs to make life liveable.

I realise as I write, that if *Burning Woman* were about facing the fear that I could be burned at the stake for doing my work and my self-expression, then *Medicine Woman* is about my fear of the institution and the System. It is my own confrontation with my greatest fear that I will be taken away, locked away, done away with, because of how my bodymind, my health, my genes are. Because I am a woman, and a sick woman. It is a deep-seated fear, and one that I have spent a lifetime trying to outrun and hide from.

The ghosts of women past haunt me – those who were drugged, institutionalised, operated on, locked up, silenced – the women I could have been, would have been… might be. I don't know when the time for this freedom of expression will be over. I am condemned by my own bodymind to a life I have no control over. To a life I would not be able to live.

This is the crux of illness – physical or mental – in being the ones who are sick: we are at the mercy of others. We are often powerless within a System that chooses how we will be treated, what we are deserving of. And that is a very scary place to be.

You and I, whose bodyminds make us vulnerable are in a position of great trust. We have to trust our lives to this System. Those who won the human lottery, who were born into a bodymind that the System considers 'normal' do not know this vulnerability.

HUSHING THE HYSTERICAL WOMAN

For generations we have been screaming,
Screaming to be heard.
For generations we have been told we were hysterical,
Eventually we fell silent.
But our bodies have kept on screaming.

In the beginning, we are told in the Christian myth of creation, was God. He created Man in his image, the first and proper human. Woman was an afterthought, an officially sanctioned helpmeet, made from his rib. The female body, with its constantly shifting hormones, menstrual cycle, risk of pregnancy, lactation, hidden sexual organs, unpredictable moods and uncontrollable sexuality has been considered a mystery: a faulty mystery cursed to suffer.

For the entirety of Western medical history, the male body has been considered the norm and the sick woman has been stuck in a bind: much of what is wrong with her has not been understood by science, it has not been studied. She is told, time and again, that there is nothing that can be done, or worse that there is in fact nothing wrong. Oftentimes her experience of her own body cannot be corroborated by existing scientific tests, or empathised with by her doctor, and is therefore disbelieved.

Many of the systemic conditions affecting women span the discrete fields that Western medicine has so nicely chopped the human being into. In a System that has divided mind from body, psyche from soma, which insists upon different specialists for each different realm, no wonder there is a lack of joined-up thinking. 'Physical' health issues are treated as more serious and real, and usually entirely separately to mental health ones, as though they exist in different countries, not the same body. When they do come together in strange and inexplicable ways, usually in the body of a woman, they are dismissed as psychosomatic. Hysterical. Which in medical parlance reads as *not real.*

From endometriosis to mental health to mesh implants, they all inform a pretty prominent narrative that women's health is not taken seriously. Not even by other women in the medical profession. Doctors just seem to assume you're a neurotic woman and probably think you're attention seeking.

TESS

As Maya Dusenbery points out in an interview, "There's this long history of viewing women as prone to hysteria. At this point, the most common term in the medical literature is 'medically unexplained symptoms.' That is a deceptively neutral term, but in medicine, it's often used to imply a psychogenic cause. Medicine's retained this idea that it can blame any symptoms it can't attribute to a physical disease on a patient's mind, and it's persistently insisted that women are especially prone to such symptoms."[81]

Our cultural tendency to dismiss the suffering of women has been written into the founding tomes of religion, medicine and history.

Men have been warned that women are not to be believed since the literal beginning of patriarchy. The first book of The Bible notes that Eve tricked Adam into taking a bite of the apple. She was cursed for her manipulation to suffer ever-more in childbirth by the Father God. And so the narrative began: a woman's suffering was justly decreed by the Creator. It was a fair punishment for her cunning and deceitful nature. Right from the beginning. Because… God says. And you can't argue with Him.

This 'knowing' has infiltrated our unconscious attitudes, regardless of our religious affiliation. Including those of medical professionals. Studies have proven time and again that women's pain is not taken as seriously as men's, and women's testimonies are generally trusted less than men's. Researchers have consistently found that "female pain is perceived as constructed or exaggerated."[82]

Rather than genuinely suffering, women have been derided as weak by their very nature. As one eighteenth century physician so beautifully describes: "Women have 'frail fibers', are easily carried away, in their idleness, by the lively movements of their imagination, are more often attacked by nervous diseases than men who are 'more robust, dried, hardened by work.'"[83]

This prejudice carries healthily on today. Women are still likely to receive less treatment until they prove that they are as sick as male patients, a phenomenon referred to in the medical community as "Yentl Syndrome."[84] According to another study: "Women report more severe levels of pain, more frequent incidences of pain, and pain of longer duration than men, but are nonetheless treated for pain less aggressively."[85] And recent research by Yale University found that many women even hesitated in seeking help for a heart attack because of concerns that they would be perceived as hypochondriacs.[86]

This is how serious the lack of belief in women's personal testimony is. This is how used women are to not being believed. This is how conditioned we have become to believing the authority of medical professionals over the evidence of our own bodyminds.

Susan Sontag digs deeper still into this tendency in her book, *Illness as Metaphor*:

Illness is interpreted as, basically, a psychological event, and people are encouraged to believe that they get sick because they (unconsciously) want to, and that they can cure themselves by the mobilization of will; that they can choose not to die of the disease. These two hypotheses are complementary. As the first seems to relieve guilt, the second reinstates it. Psychological theories of illness are a powerful means of placing the blame on the ill. Patients who are instructed that they have, unwittingly, caused their disease are also being made feel that they have deserved it.

*Some are afraid the moment I don't respond in a very simple, orthodox way. Some are immediately overly sympathetic; this can be just as annoying as the first reaction. Others are annoyed or 'let down'. It seems, to some, that my admitting being ill was like my 'giving up the fight', as though fighting it was always the way out of illness. Others were angry at my diet restrictions, my health bills, my parents' money spent on those bills. Others said I was being 'lazy' or making excuses ('Oh, don't you know how many are sick and they still go to work every day?'). Others were disbelieving, including some doctors: ('You, at your age shouldn't be this ill. And besides, you don't look ill!') This attitude was the most unhelpful. This was followed by, at my insistence that I was indeed unwell and listing – again – my symptoms, 'Well, we'll do some tests...' As though what I know about myself, my body and what is normal for me means nothing and as though I had to prove my sickness by **looking** ill. Sometimes there was a condescending doubtful tone, implying that it was 'all in my head'. I believe many women get told this and are declared inexpert on their own bodies.*

CIARA

Once our vital statistics are fine, then our illness is dismissed as being 'all in our minds'. As the only witnesses to the reality of our 'inner state' our energy levels, emotions and feeling of wellbeing, our evidence is consistently disbelieved as subjective. Because it is known that women cannot be believed. Rather than believe our own bodyminds, we are made to trust in the external explanation: that we are sick, because we are inherently weak, because of the lie "of staggering proportions that sits at the center of our lives. This lie is so pervasive that it is rendered virtually invisible. This lie is that female inferiority is the natural order, implying that all that is feminine has a natural defect."[87]

A DEPRESSING STATE OF AFFAIRS

It is a depressing state of affairs. And that is how we tend to respond. Recent studies show that almost one in four people experience depression at some point during their lives. In the past thirty years, each subsequent generation has been shown to be more likely to suffer from it.[88] According to John Geddes, professor of epidemiological psychiatry at Oxford University, "Depression is the single largest contributor to global disability that we have – a massive challenge for humankind. It affects around 350 million people worldwide and instances rose almost 20% from 2005-2015... 1 in 6 people receive proper treatment in the rich world – and 1 in 27 in the developing world."[89] In the UK the most recent research highlights the gender divide starkly: mental health problems as a whole affect more than 1 in 4 women, and fewer than 1 in 6 men.[90] According to NHS statistics for 2017-18, 1 in 6 people aged 18-64 in the UK were taking antidepressants, a quarter of whom were new users, and unsurprisingly "twice as many women are prescribed antidepressants as men, in all age groups."[91]

The World Health Organisation recognises this trend, and also the way we treat it. As they chillingly observe, "Female gender is a significant predictor of being prescribed mood altering psychotropic drugs."

The way we get women through what is expected of them in patriarchy is by medicating them.

Chicken or egg, or perhaps both, as Maya Dusenbery points out in her analysis of the way Western medicine fails women, "Studies in the 1990s suggested that as many as 30-50% of women diagnosed with depression were misdiagnosed. Furthermore, depression and anxiety are themselves symptoms of other diseases, which often go unrecognised in women. And, of course, the stress of suffering from an undiagnosed – and therefore untreated – disease often takes its mental toll. As one article points out, 'Ironically, medical misdiagnoses of physical conditions may induce depressive reactions in female patients.'"

We are not able – or willing – to take the suffering of women seriously.

....

I can't help feeling if it were men going through such symptoms they'd intervene. When it's men risking their lives with this operation, things will change. When a female billionaire or two have to have this procedure, things will change.

JANE

....

WITCHES AND MIDWIVES

When women had a place in medicine it was in a people's medicine. When that people's medicine was destroyed, there was no place for women – except in the subservient role of nurses. The set of healers who became the medical profession was distinguished not so much by its associations with modern science as by its associations with the emerging American business establishment.
Barbara Ehrenreich and Deirdre English,
Witches, Midwives and Nurses

So if male doctors and patriarchal medicine have not had a great track record of understanding and treating women's bodyminds, why haven't women just done it themselves?

Good question!

The short answer is: if we could have, we surely would have. And women throughout history have died trying to heal… and be healed.

As Barbara Ehrenreich and Deirdre English so clearly assert in their short but powerful book, *Witches, Midwives and Nurses*, "We have not been passive bystanders in the history of medicine. The present system was born in and shaped by the competition between male and female healers. The medical profession in particular is not just another institution which happens to discriminate against us: it is a fortress designed and erected to exclude us."

Women have been systematically kept from positions of power throughout the history of patriarchy. The power to heal is one of the greatest and most respected of human abilities. So, naturally, a woman did not have the natural ability… or rather could not be trusted to follow the patriarchal rules of healing.

It is certainly not that women are incapable of healing others. Women have healed. In their billions, around the world, since time immemorial in uncountable different ways: soothing the fevers of their children with cooling compresses, guiding each other through birth, healing burns and cuts in the home, giving sleeping drafts, healing herbs, ensuring that there was good nourishing food to eat, that the children were in bed in good time and their elders were close enough to the fire. They would counsel members of their community, gift amulets of strength and protection, make love with their partners, hold the hands of the dying and the shaking bodies of traumatized children. And they continue to do so, in private.

But the disappearance of women from public and prestigious healing roles within the community, and the traditional healing methods that they practised, was not due to evolution or the result of superior skills of professional male doctors or the natural rise of Western medicine based on logic and proof. It was down to systematic genocide and generations of oppression.

A 'land grab' of the healing and spiritual arts and community power was perpetrated over centuries, accompanied by violence and a propaganda campaign directed expressly by Church and State, to discredit the skills and abilities of traditional healers: medicine women, herbalists, bonesetters, wise women, clairvoyants and midwives who were burned in their hundreds of thousands as witches. The medicine women were shunned and shamed, and their communities turned against them for practising the healing arts where they in any way threatened the credibility, expertise or income of the new Medical Men.

As the practice of Western medicine was systematised, formalised, professionalised and *monetised*, women were *actively prevented* from training and practising in the State sanctioned healing sciences. When universities first began to establish faculties of medicine and professionalise healing in thirteenth century mainland Europe, women were excluded. This systematic exclusion was repeated in 1540, when King Henry VIII established surgical guilds in England.[92] The restriction held, with the occasional breach by a well-connected or well-disguised woman, until it was overturned in the New World, by Elizabeth Blackwell, the first woman to officially graduate from medical school in the US, in 1849.

But, of course that is history. Or so we thought. Just as this book was about to go to press a story broke that for over ten years, Japan's largest medical school, Tokyo Medical University, had been systematically lowering all female applicants' exam results to ensure more men became doctors, with the amount of women accepted to medical school firmly capped at 30%.[93] And it worked. Though Japan has the highest levels of female University graduates in the world, at almost 50% of the population, almost 80% of doctors are still male.[94]

Beyond Japan, any look around a modern healthcare facility will show you that women are now far better represented in medicine than in the past. In Ireland female doctors now outnumber males in the under thirty-five age bracket, reversing the dominance of male doctors for the first time.[95]

In the UK, the NHS employs 1.5 million people, putting it in the top five of the world's largest workforces[96] and 77% of these people are women.[97] But look a little closer and you will notice that just 5% of these women are doctors or dentists, as opposed to 22% of the male workforce.[98] Women, whilst having found equality as General Practitioners (family doctors) in the UK, still predominate in the lower-paid administrative and care-work roles. Only 35% of consultants[99] but a massive 89% of nurses[100] are female. Of those consultants a 2017 BBC report stated that, "On average, full-time female consultants earned nearly £14,000, or 12%, less a year than males." And "just five of the 100 highest-paid consultants in England were women, with the top-paid man earning two-and-a-half times that of the top woman."[101] In the US, Reuters report that in 2017, "male primary care doctors earned almost 18% more than their female counterparts, and men in specialities earned 36% more." And whilst African-American doctors earned $50,000 less than their white counterparts across the board, black female physicians earned $100,000 less than black male doctors.[102] And when it comes to nurses, patriarchy still most definitely rules: 91% of US nurses are female, of which 75% are white.[103]

Things are changing in the System,

But too slowly.

MEDICINE QUESTIONS

Hysterical

Have you ever been accused of being hysterical? What were the circumstances? What impact did it have on you at the time, and on your future behaviour?

Have you ever considered another woman hysterical?

How do we refer to men when they are angry or upset? Is there a gender difference in what emotions each gender is allowed to express and the words used to describe these?

How much do you know about the history of hysteria – the term and the condition? It's a fascinating subject, well-worth exploring.

Witches

Had you ever considered the connection between accusations of witchcraft and the control of women as healers before? In what ways may this have impacted your experience of women as healers, and your own abilities to heal?

HEALING ARTS

Picturing your Condition

Can you draw, paint or collage your illness or condition as it appears to you? Does it have a distinctive voice, feeling, personality or character?

What relationship do you have with it?

How are you healing or interacting with it?

What is it trying to tell you?

Which part of your body is trying to communicate most strongly?

Create – in words and images – a metaphor for your health as it is now, and how you are managing your condition and caring for your health.

What do you believe needs to happen for you to get better?

What does better look like and feel like?

BREAKDOWN

WE ARE THE CANARIES

Like the 'canary in a coal mine', our autoimmune and other chronic health conditions warn of imbalances in the world at large.
We Are Canaries.com

What if the sick women of the world, so often labelled hypochondriacs, neurotics or serial complainers, are picking up perfectly on the signs that something is wrong? What if we are registering the cultural and chemical imbalance of the modern world in our highly-sensitive bodyminds, but mistaking the main issue as being only in our own bodies, rather than the body of the world beyond us? What if we are doing what women have always done – feeling the communal pain as though it were our own – and trying to make it better?

We are told insistently that nothing is really wrong. *But it is, we know it is.* This is the cognitive dissonance we inhabit as our daily reality. This is why the constant reassurance does little to help us. This is why the medicines do not work for long. We are feeling, deep in our bones, in our nerves, in our pulse, with our powerful intuition and empathy that something is seriously wrong in the body of the world. Because it is. The research on climate change and political and economic shifts backs us up on this. But our ways of knowing are not considered valid. Our biological systems may or may not have become fully pathologised, but the signs of a sick world are quickening within us. Like creatures that can pick up the tremors of an earthquake when they are still unfelt by the human population, our highly sensitive bio-energetic systems are registering the imminent collapse of the System on which our lives depend. No wonder we are freaking out.

What makes it hard right now is that our culture does not recognise the full scale of what we are up against, nor does it see how drastically things need to shift: it thinks we can just keep papering the cracks. To believe in the demise of our culture is seen as crazy, pessimistic, deluded, paranoid, fundamentalist or invested in its destruction. How can it be collapsing when we have the internet and cell phones and airplanes and shiny hospitals and free public schooling? Our culture is obsessed with the superficial, handily ignoring the energetics that lie beneath. We are in denial that the unseen structure is fundamentally flawed: it is toxic to life.

And so when we are dismissed for what we are feeling, we learn to distrust that inner voice, our intuitive guidance, once again. We learn to turn the volume down on our inner warning system which is in direct unconscious communication with the natural world and is blaring at full volume: *Danger! Danger!*

It's just anxiety. Something wrong in your head.

But it's not. You are not just imagining it. There is not *just* something *wrong* inside *your* body or *your* brain. It is not *just you* who cannot live like this anymore. You are responding, on every level – physical, emotional, energetic – to the unique and sustained bombardment of stresses that we are all experiencing. Some of us more than others. Some of us due to our neurology or early trauma, or lack of resources are more susceptible to this stress. We are those who are sick *now*.

We are not anomalies. We are not sick individuals in a healthy context. We are the litmus test. We are the indicators of systemic illness. What we are experiencing is an autoimmune response on a species-wide scale. We have become allergic to our culture. We are infected with patriarchal symptoms which are affecting us all, starting with the most sensitive – the life-creators and nurturers – women.

....

We have embodied that which is happening with the Earth. As women we carry the grief and suffering within our bodies in order to heal it.
KERRY

....

115

I believe that whilst our bodies *are* sick – *they* are not the problem, *we* are not the problem. We are the symptoms. Of a sick culture. And whilst we need to regain our own personal wellbeing, our culture needs to heal too for us to be able to stay well.

I believe that the collapse of women's bodies and minds in the prime of life is a potential early warning of what lies ahead for our species.

In my great-grandfather's time, he and the other miners would take canaries down into the coal mines with them. Mining could release pockets of toxic gas which were invisible and unscented. Canaries were highly sensitive to this gas and would sicken and die when exposed to it. These tiny, innocent winged creatures played a vital role as a low-tech early warning system that would save miners' lives.

Like that underground gas, the danger is currently invisible to the eye, but its effects are very real.

We are the twenty-first century canaries in the coal mine.

But instead of being acknowledged as such, we are gaslighted: a term originating from the 1944 movie *Gaslight* in which a man manipulates his wife to the extent that she believes she is losing her mind.

Gaslighting is a tactic in which a person or entity, in order to gain more power, makes a victim question their reality. [...] Anyone is susceptible to gaslighting, and it is a common technique of abusers, dictators, narcissists and cult leaders. It is done slowly, so the victim doesn't realize how much they've been brainwashed.[104]

Gaslighting, the making crazy of women for what they have known but could not speak, has been the favourite tool of control for the patriarchy forever.

It is happening now. To us.

FEAR

What made you leave medicine? I asked her.

I think a better question is: what made me get into medicine? Fear. Fear of believing that I couldn't make my own creative path work. I didn't have the courage to trust my own heart. I was hard-working and found studying easy, so for my school the choices were law or medicine: drama wasn't a career option. I was also living up to the expectations of my family and being successful in their eyes held appeal for me. That was how it began… and it ended with me being hospitalised myself, after getting sick from working 100-hour weeks in the hospital.

And I wondered how many of those who are running our Establishment are in those positions because of fear: fear of failure, fear of disappointing their families or teachers, fear of not being able to make a living at what they're really passionate about, fear of making another decision when they have invested so much of their young lives and money into training, only to discover the reality of the profession as it is now. The same is true of teachers and lawyers and bankers – all those who enter the Professions, for so many reasons, only to discover a little too late the death-trap reality of the current System. I did this with teaching. Hoping to re-humanise education from the inside. But I ran for the hills when I realised how horrific the System was: for teachers and students. I knew I could not stay sane in it, it was making me sick. But many people, most people, can't or won't leave the System once they're in it, because they cannot see beyond it, because they don't have the resources, because they don't know who they are or could be beyond its definition of their worth. And so they die, slowly, trying to sustain it.

What if our current System is based on a foundation of fear that we cannot express? Fed by fear at every level. The fear of those who have to deal with it as patients, consumers or students. The fear of those working in it – that they will lose their jobs, be sued, lose a patient, be punished by their superiors if they step out of line. From the bottom to the top, there is this pervasive fear of *what if* that overrides the supposed rationality of the System.

WHY ARE WE WORKING OURSELVES TO DEATH?

One of the threads at the heart of many of our illnesses is our relationship to work. The words *wealth* and *wellness* share the same root. And so we find ourselves trying to prove our worth through work, trying to earn our place in a society that does not value or support the unproductive, a culture where death from overwork, *karoshi*, is a growing phenomenon.[105] A world where work, morality and fear are so closely woven as to be indistinguishable.

What is work and why are we in thrall to it? Firstly the formal economy is now the centre of cultural and individual life. Most things we need are no longer part of an informal economy rooted in giftwork or community labour exchange. Many of us do not have a community we can rely on, having moved away from home and the community we grew up in, with few deep-rooted social ties to call on in our time of need, we are instead reliant on the market economy to provide what we need. And to do this we need money.

But our relationship with work goes deeper. The Protestant work ethic – of work being a good and moral thing in its own right – where appearing to be busy is seen as being a better person, infiltrates Western culture, whatever your own belief system. For many the immigrant work ethic – proving yourself in a new country by working yourself half to death in order to stand on your own two feet – is a strong archetypal pull on our energy. For women there is the super-woman complex, trying to prove we can have it all. For many it is proving themselves to their families.

To heal we have to wean ourselves off these responses. It is time to uncouple work and fear. The inner fear of being judged lazy, incompetent, useless, the need to prove ourselves worthy, to compete to the death with others over scarce resources. We are human beings, but we are treated as replaceable cogs in a machine that we have no control over. But most of us are scared to change.

THE SYSTEM IS BROKEN

Growth is painful. Change is painful. But nothing is as painful as staying stuck somewhere you don't belong.
Mandy Hale

The old world is falling, but the new world isn't yet born.
Umair Haque

The System is broken, says the father on the radio angry at how his son's brain tumour was overlooked by overworked A&E staff.

The System is broken, says the TV news reporter, celebrating seventy years of the NHS, noting that there is a shortage of 100,000 nurses, a deficit of several billion pounds, and well over 4 million people waiting for operations.[106]

The System is broken, says the husband grieving his wife lost too early due to faulty cervical screening, which was covered up by authorities for years.

The System is broken, says my psychiatrist as she apologises that there is only one therapist on the public system for our area. And she only has one day a week.

The System is broken, says the co-ordinator of services of the ASD treatment facility.

The System is broken, say the teachers who cannot access the resources and support they need for their special needs students.

The System is broken, says my doctor as he apologises for the lengthy waiting lists for urgent mental health support. *And it will not be fixed in my lifetime.*

The System is broken and every day more and more are needing to access it.

The System is broken, it cannot meet our needs.

The System is broken… and it is breaking the lives of most people that come in contact with it.

All around me I see how many women are trying to navigate the health and welfare system for themselves and their families. Endlessly ploughing their energy into making the hamster wheel turn. It still seems to be women who are in the majority of doing the unpaid work of navigating bureaucracy, whose calls are answered by other under-paid, undervalued women. Figuring out how to press the right levers at the right time to get the support they need. Despite working full-time, caring full-time, barely holding their own crumbling health together.

The System is crazy-making. It is exhausting attempting to navigate the labyrinthine passages towards finding the specialists and supports you need.

I have a feeling it is designed that way so that many just give up. Women are so used to being dismissed, discredited and ignored. To not believing that they deserve help or support. Not receiving empathy. Being made to feel bad because we didn't do the right thing at the right time. We are so used to it being our fault. Because we are told, again and again, by the System that it is our fault. That it always was.

And so, it is women who are building grassroots alternatives and caring for each other. Isolated in homes through lack of social and health care, they are harnessing technology to escape their cages of silenced despair and exhaustion. It is women in the vast majority who create and populate the online health forums sharing information, hard days, lifting each other up, offering friendship and resources. Women who start support groups on the ground: a sisterhood of suffering… a suffragette sisterhood of women trying to navigate the System together, all coming to the conclusion that this is not just personal. This is political.

The System is broken, and the Master is out to lunch.

The System is broken, it is time to look beyond it.

The System is broken, it is time to create something new.

SICK AND TIRED

I am sick and tired of holding up this System with my blood, my sweat, my tears.

This broken web of white lies and turned eyes.

The pain of sustaining it is too great.

I am sick of being a woman in this culture.

Of being the magic behind the mask.

Of the energy it takes to sustain everything.

Energy that goes unvalued, unseen.

I am sick of the invisible work that happens from my hands, from my heart, from my head.

I am tired, bone tired.

I want to put the ever-rushing world on pause

Slow it down, so that I can breathe.

These bones are aching to tell me something

But I cannot hear them.

The Jenga tower of my daily life

Poised to topple, if I do not hold it up.

I am Sisyphus, pushing this family up hill.

Tomorrow I start again.

And again.

But I am no tragic hero.

I am dead tired.

However much I drop,

However much I slow down

It is never enough.

CRISIS POINT

*Illness is the shadow of Western civilisation, the antithesis of the
rampant extraversion and productivity it so values.*
Kat Duff, The Alchemy of Illness

I am not alone.

You are not alone.

There are millions of us already.

What happens when too many of us are sick? When we can't contribute financially to the world? When climate change brings ever-increasing hardship and fewer resources to go around? What then?

The wheels of capitalism cannot turn if the factories and offices aren't full of people. If we can't afford to buy what they are selling us. The wheels of capitalism cannot run when the oil runs out, when the electricity stops. Life can't carry on as normal when water is scarce, harvests fail, communities flood. What does this mean for our culture? For us as individuals? For our healthcare systems, that are already running far beyond capacity in countries where they are socialised, and are out of reach of most long-term sick, in countries where they are not? What happens when antibiotics don't work anymore? Or when too many are addicted to drugs? What happens when the length of our lives is extended but their quality has decreased? What happens when our sickness impoverishes us and our families? What happens next and does anyone care?

How can we ensure that the care of our most vulnerable humans (and those who are dedicated to caring for them) are the priority of our culture, not a thing done for profit, nor handed over to charities, not skimped on or ignored? How can we share the burden of care?

These are the questions that our governments are evading. These are the answers that our exhausted communities are having to try to create answers to with little support. This is where we are having to get creative at the grassroots.

Because at the moment it falls to the individual, it falls to the shattered nuclear family, to charities. Everyone else is too busy just trying to survive themselves, the pace of life is too fast, the need to earn enough to get by is taking all our time and energy, and our communities have disintegrated under the pressures of efficiency.

But even so, we have not, in our government's eyes reached full crisis point. And so little action is being taken from on high. They have bigger priorities... like nuclear weapons.

Crisis and emergency are written into the core of Western culture as the main response to imbalance and need. Our governments go from years of paralysis and procrastination – see climate change, Brexit, North Korea, Syria – to leaping to all-out war and a state of emergency in order to mobilise the money, human resources and energy they need to accomplish something.

Wrapped up in the Western medical approach to health is this emergency mindset: ignore the early symptoms, then big daddy steps in with his 'invisible hand' and sorts out the mess aggressively, reasserting his dominance, which is often deeply costly – both financially and traumatically.

This modus operandi communicates an extreme powerlessness to all those involved – those that have been running on limited resources, who have been asking for the necessary support, supplies and assistance, who have been denied them consistently are suddenly depicted as weak and out of control, not doing their job when the authorities step in. We see this played out again and again across the board in government services.

We have reached crisis point. As individuals. As cultures.

The Chinese character for crisis combines danger and opportunity. We are at the stage where it is still within our power to choose which it will be. Just.

We are inhabiting the time of the great disruption. The great awakening. Where that which has gone before can no longer lead us. We are looking for new ways forward. Ways to not just survive but to thrive.

Patriarchy, as seen in its current form within Western capitalism and corporate culture, has shown itself to be incompatible with life itself. The contradictions are becoming harder to bear and we are personally embodying the stresses of an unsustainable collective culture. But we do not see the connection between our individual broken systems, and the broken System. We do not connect the autoimmune response in our bodies, and the autoimmune response within humanity as we turn on our own kind. We do not see the connection between our cultural climate change and our inner climate change, the outer burnout of unsustainable energy being reflected by inner burnout, the cultural anxiety and our inner anxiety, economic depression and personal depression. We do not see, because we have not been taught to see this way. We have not been raised with an intuitive understanding of Systems Theory, or an environmental or spiritual knowing of our innate interconnectedness.

The problems we are facing are multiple and systemic. But they are not being dealt with on this level. Instead they are being treated as individual problems on an emergency basis.

The habitual patriarchal response to threat and change is to fight, to declare war. And so we find that we are fighting wars on every level – against climate change and terrorism and cancer and depression and drugs. The man-made, heroic battle of dominance over nature is being played out in our bodies. And we find that we are on the losing side… against ourselves.

This endless war is not working. We are not winning. We are so tired of fighting. But still we keep on being told that we must act the hero. Throwing all our financial and emotional resources at this war on life. Working ourselves to death.

We are scared of the come down from the constant buzz of adrenaline that we have learned to live under. Scared of having to face the fear and the pain we have been drugging with our stress and busyness. Scared of what lies on the other side.

We have been running from this moment for a long time.

It was well over a hundred years ago that those with their finger on the pulse of their culture started to remark that Western civilization was sick and dying: George Orwell, D.H. Lawrence, Virginia Woolf and T. S. Eliot to name a few. The heroic myth, so long pushed by science and colonialism, of our culture reaching ever-greater heights, was being questioned back then. From the inside. By privileged white folk who benefited most from its success.

Our culture is crumbling faster now. Western patriarchy is dying. And it's taking us down with it.

"The pain you feel," says Joe Brewer in a powerful blog post, "is capitalism dying."[107] Or as Tracy Evans says, "These are the death throes of patriarchy, love. This is what it feels like."

We are trying to stay alive in the midst of a dying culture.

The story we have seen on our screens *ad nauseum* is that the hero will save us, at the eleventh hour, and all will be happily-ever-after.

All we have to do is cry out, and he will save us.

PANIC BUTTON

For years I have tried to manage alone.
Scared of what happened when I pressed the panic button.
Scared that I would lose control as everyone came running
To take my life out of my hands whilst they cared for me.
One day, when I could no longer cope alone,
I pressed the panic button.
Expecting the suspicious saviours to come running.
But. Nothing. Happened.
I pressed it again.
No one came.
Again. Again.
Nothing. No one.
I learned that in this culture on fire,
In this life on fire,
I was the fire warden:
The doctors were all out sick.
Medicine Woman was the only one on call.
But I didn't have her number,
And no address either.
The flames rose,
The panic rose,
The smoke rose,
Darkness fell.
The panic button wailed in the darkness.
Still no one came.

MEDICINE QUESTIONS

Crisis

What experience have you had of crisis in the past?

Have you experienced it as a time of danger and opportunity?

What strengths did you develop as a result of it?

What traumas do you still carry from it?

What symptoms of cultural systemic collapse can you see around you?

Are there ways that you can see equivalent system collapses in your own family?

Can you recognise systemic collapse in your own body? Have you ever considered that they might be related, if so how? If not, can you begin to see the connections now? How do you feel about this?

Panic Button

Have you ever had to press a panic button – literal or metaphorical? Tell your story of what happened when you did… and what you were expecting would happen.

The System

How do you see or understand the System? What is your relationship with it? How much power do you feel you have within it?

How has your faith/confidence in yourself, and in the System, been changed by your experiences?

How much energy do you put into engaging with or fighting the System? Are there other ways you would prefer to use this energy? How could you use it to achieve other results to support yourself or your family?

Do you agree with my assertion that "the System is broken"?

How have your interactions with the System affected your health?

What parallels can you see between the sickness in your own body, in your family, in your community, in your culture and in the natural world?

How much of yourself is invested in our current culture: your financial assets, identity, family history? How much do you have to lose? How hard will you fight to retain what is being lost?

What is the story that our culture is telling you about your sickness? Why are you sick? How can you heal?

What is our culture telling you about your value as a person when sick? When well?

How much power do you hold in this story?

What vision do you have of how things could be different?

What is your relationship with change? Does it scare you? How hard do you tend to resist change?

What has your previous experience of cultural change been – does it hold any trauma for you or your lineage?

What might lie beyond the System? How can you access it, connect with it or help to strengthen it?

Have you been told about the options available to you outside the System?

Has a lack of money delayed or prevented you from accessing a doctor /hospital/alternative health?

What is your attitude to alternative health? What has influenced this?

What is your doctor's attitude to alternative medicine?

What is your family's attitude to alternative medicine?

Where do you source your information from? Why do you trust this source?

How do you establish what sources of healing or information are trustworthy? How did you learn this?

HEALING ARTS

The System

Can you create an image of the System? Is it like an old-fashioned machine full of cogs and levers? Or is it a more modern version, for example a circuit board? Is it more like a city or an Underground train map? Is it a series of labelled boxes? What role do people have in this System? What is their relationship with it? Where are you in the System? How can you depict yourself? Within this understanding of the System how might you (metaphorically) effect change?

The Canary in the Coalmine

What does the image of the canary in the coalmine mean to you? Is it a metaphor you are familiar with? Do you identify with it in terms of your own experience?

I invite you to do a WORD+image piece, collage, art work or piece of writing on this metaphor. How can you depict the darkness of the mine, the silent threat of the unseen gas, the hardworking men risking their lives, the role of the canary caged, just there to sing in the darkness and die? Do you identify with the experience of being a caged bird, the metaphor of the feathered being with wings that has been deprived of freedom? As you work on this creative piece or meditate on the image consider: what does the image of the songbird represent for you? What does the cage represent? Is there a miner who you have been a guardian for, trying to protect with your own life? Can you free the bird? What happens if you open the cage? What does freedom look like? How can it be achieved? How else can you use your voice and wings to help serve and save humanity rather than sacrificing your life?

Look again at the metaphor of mining, of entering the underworld looking for things of value. Can you see that this is what you are doing as you explore the healing process, as you engage with your unconscious psychic* material?

Gaslighting

When in your life have you experienced gaslighting? How long did it take you to realise that this was happening? How did you realise? What had to change before you could release yourself from the situation? How did you?

For me, putting together the pieces of the canary in the coal mine and the idea of gaslighting was a major aha! moment. Is this connection meaningful to you? I invite you to do a WORD+image piece, collage, art work or piece of writing on this metaphor or the connection between them.

RELEASING THE NEGATIVE FEMININE ARCHETYPES OF HEROIC MEDICINE

SOMEONE SAVE ME

The narrative of healing that we have been immersed in since childhood is the myth of the hero: the founding myth of patriarchy, where the brave and worthy man wages war to save humanity from the darkness, be it foreign invaders, terrifying monsters, natural disasters or deadly viruses, in a prolonged war of righteousness versus evil. Woman has been demoted to 'she who must be saved' – victim, patient or sexy damsel in distress, depending on her worthiness and waist size. We can see this story played out from the Bible through to the Hollywood movies of today. And just a glance at any newspaper will confirm to you that this is the frame of reference that we overlay onto our daily realities and moments of history too: one has to be Hero, or one is Victim.

So at first we might try to be our own heroes, having imbibed the message of equality. We shrug off the pain, grit our teeth, firm up our bodies and push through: no pain, no gain we are told. We did not realise that we would never make the grade: women can never be the Heroes within patriarchy. Our ultimate role, as women, is prescribed: Victim.

Whilst we may initially resist the demotion from our hard-won and patriarchal-approved Good Girl roles of good wife, good mother, good worker, we discover, as illness draws on sapping the last of our energy, the sweet relief of finally being able to off-load our overwhelming adult female burden. As we realise that we are unable to 'save' ourselves, we begin, like abandoned children, to look longingly for a hero outside. We long for daddy to see our suffering and save us.

Within the System doctors and priests have been socialised to take on the role of father figure – some embody the benign caring father, others the authoritarian dictator. Nurses and receptionists take on the mother role of caring and nagging. And so a psychological dynamic is set up. The sick woman becomes child-like, the mother's unconditional love is longed for but instead she is treated with the detached objectivity of the professional father.

It is not surprising therefore to find that in times of suffering we are psychologically transported back to ways of being that we learned the first time we felt weak and helpless. When this inner child comes to the fore, she brings with her the cobwebs and shadows of our inner selves that we have long ignored, denied or neglected. She brings with her memories of how we were cared for – or not – as children. Sickness summons forth the spectre of the scared, lonely, vulnerable child who projects her unconscious childhood needs onto those who she comes into contact with now – partners, healthcare workers, children and friends. She projects onto them the all-powerful mother or father figure she experienced or longed for. Or she shuts herself off from them, as she has learned to, if previous caregivers were unreliable.

If and when the care doesn't come from our broken System, our state sponsored parents, the feeling of abandonment, rejection, hurt and anger builds.

Nobody cares.

Why does nobody care about me?

I DESERVE TO SUFFER

When we are not met in our pain, when our calls for help are not answered, this may trigger another belief that many of us have acquired along the way, either ingrained through a religious upbringing, poor attachment to carers, abuse or a lack of self-worth: we deserve to suffer. We may think that we deserve to suffer because we are worthless or inherently bad, because we are undeserving of love, because we don't look after ourselves well enough, we don't eat properly, or perhaps that we are not worth treating. We may not feel we deserve to spend the money or the time on ourselves that we need to heal.

As sick people we have to constantly engage with this Victim identity, in our own heads and in the world, as we feel ourselves disempowered, depressed, punished by others, abandoned, lonely, hurt and resentful of a culture and System that makes many demands of us but treats us without the dignity we deserve when we suffer: a culture that doesn't care.

We live in a culture of victim blaming and shaming. It's much easier to ignore or blame the sufferer than to help fix their problems and face the shadows in our world and ourselves that we would rather avoid. Victim blaming takes the issue out of society's hands and passes it, like a hot potato, back to the person with the problem.

Along with victim blaming often comes that issue we've discussed many times already – disbelief. Choosing to believe the person in the position of Systemic power and to disbelieve the woman, the victim. Choosing to place the blame for suffering firmly with the sufferer. The more invisible the illness – as with mental health and autoimmune conditions – the easier it is to do this.

You see, there is, and always has been, a careful connection made in patriarchy between morality and health. The ideal in our culture is to be the beautiful, wealthy, healthy person, the upholder of the heroic story, the liver of the American dream. So in a culture that does not acknowledge its own complicity in every level of our illness, the blame for illness again can be firmly laid at the feet of the individual: they are the loser, the weak one, the victim. They are in need of our pity or our disgust.

....

I often ask what great offense I committed in a past life to deserve what caused my PTSD. I don't know if I really believe it was some kind of karmic retribution. But I think it's human to search for reasons why. I tend to react bitterly when people talk about it like it was some great lesson from the universe. Something to learn and grow from. I think it's pretty easy to put that spin on it when it happens to you. I think people have a tendency to make light of 'invisible illnesses'. I try really hard to make an effort to be a positive person. But I still feel like I'm being punished.
MELISSA

....

Our Western medical model seeks to sustain this narrative of victim-hood and disempowerment by classing the injured and the ill as victims. This is a narrative which informs how we treat the ill, and how we feel about ourselves when we are sick. We are neither explicitly taught nor supported in our culture how to navigate illness, physical or mental decline or change as an integral part of moving through life, precisely because illness is seen as degenerate, sinister, a threatening other state of being to be avoided. We are not shown how to move through illness internally, how to assimilate its changes or how to engage spiritually with it. We are merely taught to avoid it, and to fight it: to resist change at all costs.

And if we don't or we can't, we are its victims, in a culture that wants heroes.

....

The moment I start sliding back into victim mode I almost instantaneously experience a flare-up of some sort. However, I do struggle with others' perception of my health struggles. I'm still probing why, but if someone doesn't understand the extent of what I've experienced, or they dramatise it, I feel very triggered. So I suppose there is something in there about 'owning' it, about it being 'mine', rather than simply part of a universal experience we all share in some degree.

ZOË

....

As women we have been taught to be victims by our culture. We have been consistently disempowered. We have consistently learned that we cannot advocate for our needs, that we should put others ahead of ourselves. Eventually after more suffering than we can handle, after experiencing our powerlessness more times than our spirit can bear, we agree to our place in the heroic narrative. We *believe* ourselves to be Victims.

SICKNESS STEALS

Sickness steals
My body, my energy, my mind.
She steals my future, my certainty, my past.
She takes my trust, my voice,
My life.
This life that scares me so much,
That I have valued so little,
Still I treat it like a newborn bird.
Sickness steals all this
And leaves me here alone
Hostage to her demands.
I must reclaim each facet of myself from her hands,
Fight for my life,
Take a stand for this self that I never was too sure about
For this body, this mind.
To claim them as my own.
At last.
The prize I always had but never truly wanted
Becomes the thing I will die trying to reclaim.
This life which time and again I have
Dismissed, despaired of, overlooked, bemoaned.
Will you fight for it now? she asks.

THE VICTIM AND THE CRAZY WOMAN

After being victimised for so long by the System, we may discover that
the Victim has her own shadow power: she can command the sympathy of others. After so long of not being believed, of not being seen or
heard, of losing our identity to our sickness, it may be wonderfully re-
freshing to finally find a way to be cared for by others. But when their

attention or dedication begin to wane, we discover that this caring can only be attained by dramatising or constantly reasserting our needs.

The Victim is one who does not have access to nor outlet for her righteous fury at her treatment as 'less than'. She is one who has learned to turn the harm on herself, to get sympathy and attention for her woundedness, rather than to release the pain and suffering that has been wrought on her and finally to alchemise it into her own power. She is the one who sticks with the old story because it still holds power over her. It is easier, more familiar, for her to suffer, than to demand that others make amends or change. It is easier to blame than forgive. Easier to stay stuck than risk freedom.

Embodying the archetype of Victim means we do not need to fully articulate our needs or attempt to meet them, but instead can manipulate others using guilt as a currency. We can learn to drain others' pity and attention from them as our own second-hand energy, to replace that which we do not have ourselves. We may believe from our experiences that we are unworthy of care or love unless it is earned in an emotional trade off. We may believe we have no real power of our own. This learned helplessness was, for many of us, a valid and valuable survival technique.

But the Victim can become a fixed identity – a dominant and defining shadow self rather than just one of a larger cast of characters. We may over time invest the majority of our energy into the persona of the Victim. We may begin to attach to and need to assert ourselves almost solely through the lens of our illness in order to gain control, sympathy or power. In a culture that denies and sabotages self-advocacy, self-care and self-awareness in women, this is perhaps an inevitability. Our status as sufferer may bring with it membership of certain groups and a feeling of belonging, that we risk losing if we recover. And so we may begin to identify ourselves with our illness to the exclusion of any other identity, interacting only with other wounded folk in what Caroline Myss calls "the language of wounds": focusing on our victimhood as our sole identity. For women who have historically been excluded from much of mainstream culture, who have been disbelieved and uncared for, who have on every level felt the pain of not belonging, it is completely understandable.

There is a subtle but crucial difference between a community of healing, and a community of sickness. Often our healing can be taken as a slight or personal affront to those who are still sick. They may feel abandoned, hurt, or as though you weren't really sick, or angry as to why they are still.

As Victims we may believe the lie that we are powerless to affect change. We feel trapped by horror and suffering not of our own making. We have smiled and bitten our tongues and stayed silent so many times so as not to bring greater danger on ourselves. Our silence and submission were a valid survival mechanism. But not anymore. Because the suffering is too big, the suffering that we have learned to consume for others is now consuming us.

To enter the healing ground we have to renounce victimhood, break our silence and reclaim our power: our right and our ability to heal and the possibility of transformation.

We have been cast as victims of patriarchal culture. But we are not Victims.

Our brains are not failing. Our bodies are not flawed. Our unconsciousness is merely emerging at last. We can no longer suppress our knowing because it does not fit with their model of reality. We have to learn to believe the evidence of our own bodyminds at last. To know that we are not crazy. Not in the way they may accuse us, or that we fear we may be. It is the model that is broken. Not us. We are being stretched to our limits trying to sustain its demands and pretence.

As women we have been defined for too long by others, for our lack, our weakness, for all that we were too much of or not enough of. It is time for us to take back the power of naming. To know that we are not our brokenness. Our illness is a vital stage of our inner transformation but it is not our everything.

In these transition times we are learning to embody the archetype of the Crazy Woman – she who can see, feel, know beyond the box of the patriarchal paradigm. We are having to acknowledge – at last – our knowing, deep in our bones, of the truth that they deny.

The branches of the medical establishment are deeply entwined within the patriarchal Establishment, and they have no interest in relinquishing the power, profit or privilege that goes with this any time soon.

But the roots to a different sort of medicine are there, they go deep down into our heritage as women, into so many native heritages, into our human heritage. In the roots lies our potential to heal, we simply need to reconnect to them.

MEDICINE QUESTIONS

Victim

In what ways have you been treated like a victim? In what ways do you act like one? How and why did you first learn to do this?

Can you acknowledge how you get your needs met by playing the Victim? How do you access what you are too scared to ask for in other ways? What support do you need that you do not feel you can ask for?

How might you begin to express these needs to others in healthier ways – perhaps writing an email or a letter? Searching for support? How might you meet some of these needs yourself?

How much does being the Victim help you to offload your responsibilities to others?

How do you, in the words of Caroline Myss, "speak from your wounds"? How do you identify with them? How do you identify with others through your woundedness?

Who would you be without your sickness? What would you lose if you were no longer sick? Are you willing or prepared to sacrifice this? How else could you get this need to belong and be seen met?

What identity do you have beyond your woundedness? How else would you like to define yourself? How would you like others to perceive this greater reality of you?

How can you transmute and shift the energy within you… so that your history, your pain does not become your defining quality? Is there a ceremony you would like to create, or some bodywork that might help to shift the energy from your body?

Victim/Saviour

Create an image of yourself as victim. Who is victimising you – can you make an image of them? Who is your saviour? Make an image of them too. Now make an image of yourself as powerful – keep this somewhere where you can see it.

Healing Allies

The role of the healing ally should ideally be a partnership of expertise, another pair of hands, eyes, heart and mind to help us to see what we are blind to – physically or emotionally, to help us hear the messages we may be deaf to, to provide medicine that we cannot access ourselves and to support us as we make health-making changes in our relationships with our bodies.

What does the term 'healing ally' mean to you?

Do you feel your current doctor is: an ally, partner, expert, authority, fit for purpose? What is needed to improve?

What healing allies are you still searching for? Can you put into words the qualities you would like them to have?

Can you make an image of the healing ally you are longing for?

ANOTHER WAY

THE MISSING LINK

There are more things in heaven and earth, Horatio,
Than are dreamt of in your philosophy.
William Shakespeare, *Hamlet*

Our official knowing about ourselves is partial – it has stopped at the level of the masculine rational mind. Our scientific research has been limited and curtailed by financial, gendered, racial and political patriarchal prejudice and belief. Science as it is currently and has been historically carried out, is not the independent, purely rational or objective practice it purports to be. Much is dismissed out of hand because it doesn't sit right within the scientific paradigm. This neither negates the existence nor the value or importance of the 'other'.

The focus of science thus far has been on the material plane, our physics based on a Newtonian understanding of the universe. The metaphysical – the realm of psyche, soul, energy and ideas – has been sidelined, left to those who have been dismissed as crackpots, quacks, cranks and crazies. And some are. Just as some scientists have been. But the need for our metaphysics to reconnect with our physical sciences is long overdue.

In the late nineteenth and early twentieth centuries, many groups and individuals endeavoured to heal this split – but much of their work became more about the performance of the unseen through mediumship, séance and magic, in order to earn a living, power, prestige, or influence. Through the work of theosophists, hypnotists, quantum physicists and the father of analytical psychology C.G. Jung our understanding of the unseen realms of energy was growing. But two

World Wars shut down this growth of alternative knowledge, channelling it into the service of war – creating nuclear bombs with the energetic manipulations discovered by quantum physics and CIA uses of psychological warfare.

This hunger for a broader understanding of reality came again after the recovery from World War Two through the hippie movement in the 1960s and 1970s – but this time it was more deeply counter-cultural, more detached from science. As Westerners began travelling to new cultures, especially in Asia, they developed an awareness of other healing systems beyond their own, but more ancient, which offered valid health-care alternatives to large populations, systems such as: yoga, Ayurveda and Chinese medicine. They also began to rediscover and develop Western alternatives: herbalism, homeopathy, Alexander technique, biofeedback...

But the two sides – mainstream and alternative – have become two tribes, engaged in a protracted turf war over whose view of reality is correct, warring ideologues and financial competitors, rather than potentially complimentary and collaborative ways of understanding ourselves and our world more fully.

TURF WAR

There are no rules – no how to heal,
No right or wrong – no how to feel.
Anon

As more and more people have become disillusioned with Western medicine and its fixation on pathology – the science of the causes and effects of diseases – rather than on what creates and maintains *health*, the previously niche fields of alternative medicine have moved further into the mainstream.

But rather than admitting this reality, the System continues its insistence there is only one right way to heal, one real understanding, and that is *their* way: the scientific method and Western medicine has it all covered. Their cure is just around the corner. And anything that isn't covered by their science doesn't really matter. Doesn't really count. Is just plain stupid. Unless *they* can brand and monetise, regulate and control it. Unless they can explain it logically they will not consider it as valid, nor integrate it into approved healing practices.

....

Because Western medicine is very limited, in my case, I don't feel like I have to choose between that and alternative approaches. In some ways, the alternatives have been my only option, and they are certainly what I feel more drawn to. That said, I've had little or no success with most of the treatments I have tried – though I am sure that the accumulation of many things over time has helped. Still, I'd say that the natural approach has yielded more results and I cannot be without certain supplements.
I find that I go to see my doctor mainly to update him on my situation, and occasionally when I need tests done, but not so much for 'treatments'. In fact, I avoid my doctor as much as possible, and wish that I didn't have to rely on him for testing, as it would be more helpful if other people, who are more knowledgeable about my situation, were the ones directing that. It is those other people who provide the treatments, or I just potter along on my own.
I see the benefit of Western medicine in certain areas, but am generally a little sceptical about it. It is often wonderful for serious or distinct problems, but very ineffective when it comes to CFS, because it is not well understood, and treatments are few. Thus, my focus is on the alternative and holistic approach – body, mind and spirit – something that I am still finding ways to explore and work on. Frustratingly, I am doing most of the work on my own. I've bounced around a lot over the years, trying one thing, then another. When that doesn't work, getting a bit down about it for a while; then becoming desperate again, or newly motivated, and trying something else; then having that not work, and so on.
I'm stubborn, and therefore won't just give up, but I think I need an approach that covers all the bases, and have not found anyone who could provide me with that. Thus, I need both Western medicine (testing and certain medical supplements) and alternative fields, working together, yet haven't found a way to combine the two.
THERESE

....

Women in particular are hungry for more and better when it comes to healthcare, having been failed by Western medicine for chronic conditions for so long. A 2015 study of 35,000 Americans noted that women made up 60% of users of complementary and alternative (CAM) health users and were more likely to use more than one modality.[108] Thirty to thirty-five per cent of women used complementary or alternative health in the last twelve months, a statistic which has stayed steady since its massive growth in the 1990s. It is also no coincidence that there is a far higher prevalence of female practitioners within these alternative fields.[109] Women are finding ways to heal that Western medicine has denied exist. These are women who are not finding their health cared for within the System, who are looking beyond it. These practitioners are women who are not able to provide the healthcare that women need under the aegis of the System and are finding other ways to care for women outside of it.

But the media and medical professionals often like to paint alternative health practices as irrational, and those who use them as crazy. Yes, we're back to the good old hysterical women stereotype.

This was really brought into focus for me as I read a review of one (male) scientist's angry book in a UK broadsheet's literary supplement. The author's bile was firmly focused on those who dismiss Western science and follow what he believes to be quackery. As I read I noticed something unremarked upon by the reviewer, also a man: of the nine examples of gullible folks using crazy cures and rejecting advanced medicine Every. Single. One. was a woman. All these women were sick. They weren't finding the cures they needed within the Western pharmaceutical model. They were tired of being disbelieved, tired of suffering… and so they were looking for hope, care, comfort and potential healing somewhere else. *But Western medicine is the only way!* yell these men, *Only these women are too stupid to see it!*

But this is simply not true. According to the 2015 study, "Compared to male CAM users, female CAM users were more likely to have a Bachelor degree, to be divorced/separated or widowed, and less likely to earn $75,000 or more." So these aren't rich women with money to burn and they aren't stupid women. They are women who have been highly educated within our System and are being led by their own brains and bodies to look beyond it. They are women who know that they are not being seen or understood by the System and are sick and tired of it.

This makes the Establishment very uncomfortable. The fact that many alternative modes of healing operate outside of the grasp of the scientific world view makes them dangerously heretical: they do not adhere to the agreed cultural dogma so they must be controlled. And so state regulations seek to limit the practices of homeopathy, the availability of herbal medicines, the practice of midwives, research funding is limited and any research that is done is rounded on. And on the ground medical professionals use their scepticism to scare women away from these alternative routes.

We have reached a point where ever-growing numbers of women are sick and do not trust the System. The medical profession disbelieves the reality of their sickness. But the tide is turning. The balance of power is shifting, as women in ever-larger numbers are now disbelieving the System that has disbelieved them for so long.

Where once there was a turf war between Church and science over the care (and profit) of our bodies and souls, a new turf war is now firmly entrenched between the medical establishment and the alternative health community, between the patriarchal system and the chronically sick women of the world, who are, once again stuck in the schism, in no-man's land.

NO MAN'S LAND

I believe that the modern medical preference for drugs and surgery as treatments is part of the aggressive patriarchal approach to disease. That which is natural and nontoxic is seen as inferior to the 'big guns' of drugs.
Dr Christiane Northrup,
Women's Bodies, Women's Wisdom

There is still, in these supposedly tolerant times, a shaming that falls on those whom the System cannot help, those who in their desperation to heal have to venture outside the current paradigm, whilst those who are comfortably cared for by the System exist happily in their bubbles, interacting with others in the bubble, speaking a different language.

We see it not just in medicine but in law, politics, policing: the aghast looks of the Establishment who do not understand this populist revolt against the current culture which is very cosy for them. Often the results are a knee-jerk reaction against the Establishment – as we saw with Brexit and the Trump election – an over-simplification of the facts fed by those who want to shake things up for ego-kicks and personal gain, to those who long for change as a long-overdue medicine for their individual sense of powerlessness and who long for better for their families and communities.

Those for whom the System works are exasperated, exercised by the credulity and the idiocy of those who try other ways, not understanding that if they were in the same situation, they would most likely be doing the same. Stepping outside of the System can be scary – we no longer know who or what can be trusted. But we know, through long wearying experience, that the System is not working for us. And so we have no choice but to look elsewhere: our survival instinct is strong.

Whilst the fact that the overriding arrogance of patriarchal institutions is no longer being tolerated in the same way it was can only be a good thing, with this rejection of the 'bad' also comes a wholesale rejection of much of the good: the carefully researched and painstakingly studied; professional expertise; dedicated work and historical precedence in preference for hearsay, gut feeling and trusting friends or dodgy online articles.

And so here we are. In uncharted territory in almost every area of our lives. In a post-truth world without any absolutes and lots of conflicting opinions and fake news… We could panic. We could look to someone to save us. Or we could help to find new ways forward, based on both knowledge and wisdom… if we are brave enough to try.

SCATTERED PIECES

We find ourselves with an incomplete map of what it means to be human. Western science has carefully charted the physical body over centuries. But the bit of the map showing the non-material parts of the person was ripped to shreds and thrown to the wind in the wake of the Enlightenment.

Many of us in the West are now running after those pieces, trying to put them back together. However in the meantime, the world around us has changed since native cultures first developed their more holistic maps of what it meant to be human. Parts are the same, of course, but much is different. New technology, chemicals, urban environments, climate patterns, family and community structures, foods, gender identities, new illnesses, less wilderness and far larger global populations are changing what it means to be human on a fundamental level.

We cannot go back. We must find new ways forward. New maps that incorporate the ancient and the modern territories of the human bodymind and soul, that can exist in the world we inhabit today.

Because it wasn't just a paper map that was torn in two but our inner psychic map: the paradigm that guides our knowing about ourselves and our world, which navigates our steps and informs our decisions. Without it we are lost.

Our philosophical schism has been internalised and embodied. To heal, to survive, we have to expand our perspective of what is true and who we are. We have to see and name reality in newer, fuller ways. We need to consciously admit to ourselves and each other the change that we are inhabiting, to release the psychic pressure of cognitive dissonance which is freezing our bodyminds with fear, depressing our creative responses to this healing crisis.

PARADIGM SHIFT

*When enough significant anomalies have accrued against a current paradigm, the scientific discipline is thrown into a state of **crisis**, according to Kuhn. During this crisis, new ideas, perhaps ones previously discarded, are tried. Eventually a **new** paradigm is formed, which gains its own new followers, and an intellectual 'battle' takes place between the followers of the new paradigm and the hold-outs of the old paradigm.[110]*

This is where we are right now. Both blessed and cursed to be inhabiting perhaps the most significant paradigm shift in our history as a species.

But we must be careful, as we emerge from the old paradigm, that we do not unconsciously get drawn back into its mirror image.

If we do not learn to recognise the structures of patriarchy within Western medicine and within ourselves, we can fall just as trustingly into its web in a culture that is not our own. When we are used to the dynamic of handing over our power to a paternal authority, it does not matter if he is in a business suit or wears saffron robes, whether she heals with ancient Chinese medicine or modern pharmaceuticals. If we enter the world of alternative medicine with the same longing for salvation that we have been taught by our culture, we will experience the same dynamic, whatever the medicine path we follow.

This is why it is important to move from the artificial schism of our cultural narrative, from the mentality of 'Western medicine bad, all alternatives good' to being able to engage critically with any healing tradition we use, learning how to research well, find reliable trustworthy sources, hone our instincts, and stay centred in our own power. We must learn how to work in partnership with our healing allies, whoever they may be.

It is time to move, not just as individuals, but as a culture from this either/or mentality, this war between enemy factions, fighting for power, money and control, to a healing partnership for the good of all.

WHAT COMES NEXT?

We are moving into the twenty-first century on a sick planet. This is a new situation requiring not just an expansion of consciousness but a mutation of consciousness.
Marion Woodman, *Leaving My Father's House*

Sickness or systemic collapse is not part of the American Dream so central to our heroic myth. It was never part of the plan. But life is, as John Lennon sagely remarked, what happens when we're busy making other plans.

Life is showing us that reality is far more complex, mysterious and irrational than we have allowed for within our cultural narrative. We are not in control of its forces.

Patriarchy, it turns out, is only a small story that we have been telling ourselves. Much of importance has been omitted or overlooked from the narrative we have inhabited. Life is far bigger than our map allows for. Things must change, and fast, if we as individuals and a species want to continue much longer.

What we are currently suffering from is a multi-dimensional sickness of all our personal systems – on a physical, mental, energetic and soul level. We are also experiencing this on a cultural level. Furthermore our bodyminds are registering not only the current imbalances of our personal and collective systems, but also processing the results of centuries of unacknowledged and unexpressed imbalance, which have been buried in silence and fear. And our current suffering is in turn impacting the development and health of the generations being born and raised now, and those yet to be born. The crisis we are in calls for healing on levels and dimensions that humanity has never previously had to deal with.

This is the size of the crisis that no one currently in power will dare admit. Because they cannot or will not.

The time for denial is over.

If patriarchy has been a collective trance, a limited dream state within narrow parameters, we are waking up to the fullness of possibility that lies beyond it. But if patriarchy is both our conditioned mental structure and also our physical structure – if it is what has bound and contained us, how can we see it for what it is, clearly, objectively? If this is the end of patriarchy – what happens next? Can we survive it? Can we thrive beyond it? Or will it take us all down?

We are still only part way down the road. But the brakes are off and we're hurtling downhill. The blind corners are coming fast, and as we've seen, the statistics for diagnosis of so many chronic illnesses are rising at unprecedented rates. In living systems crises are not insular events: one impacts and exacerbates another – just as high winds fan the flames of individual forest fires, joining them up. Climate change causes not just warmer air temperatures but rising sea levels and erratic weather patterns. Cancer in one part of the body spreads easily to other parts causing further complications. Mental health issues in one member of a family impact the whole family's health. We are having to acknowledge that illness is systemic – not just within discrete individual bodies, but within our communities. We are not machines but part of a living, highly complex interconnected eco-system.

We are remembering, at last, who we are.

Our mission now is not to revert to superstition and dogmatic control, rejecting and refusing any sign of technological advance. But rather to integrate the incredible gifts and gains that science has brought us, whilst reconnecting to what makes us human as well. Can what was unconscious and instinctive for the first two hundred thousand years of humanity, be consciously regained and reintegrated with our technological advancement? Can our humanity be healed?

ENOUGH!

Enough!

I have had enough.

I long for answers. For a new story. I yearn for healing. I long for Medicine Woman – a medicine woman – perhaps more than I have yearned for anything or anyone in my whole life. I yearn for someone with whom I can take the journey. Someone who can navigate the complexity of my being, speak in the language of dreams and paint and silence, who can untangle trauma like knitting wool. Someone who can read my body and know what nutrients it is lacking, where its weaknesses lie, where infection has set in.

I need someone who knows me. Who I get for more than ten minutes. Who doesn't spend more time reading my notes, than reading me. I need someone who remembers my story. Who will take my suffering as seriously as I do, to whom my healing matters as much as it does to me. Someone to walk with me as I learn the ways of my bodymind and soul.

I long for she with whom I feel safe. She who I can trust completely. My body needs her caring, my soul keens for her wisdom, to be witnessed in my vulnerability and not be judged defective. To be accepted as I am.

I long for the Medicine Woman who can awaken the medicine woman within me.

I search for her traces as I walk the hospital corridors – polished and windowless, lined with machines that go beep, trolleys of patients, the smell of cabbage and antiseptic – plastic and shining metal and strip lights as far as the eye can see. I wonder…

Where can the soul reside in this place of sick bodies? Where is the Medicine Woman? How can we let her in? Is there space for her sooth-ing hand and listening ear amongst these mountains of medical notes and forms in triplicate? Is she here in the noisy night filled with nurses' rounds and medication trolleys when healing rest is needed?

Where is she?

I'm sick and tired of half answers for the bedridden sisters around the world. The white-washing of their experience. The silencing of their symptoms. Their systems broken into little boxes to be ticked by the System.

Our bodies speak, if you would only listen. They speak another lan-guage: the mother tongue.

It's half the puzzle, the missing pieces you have been searching for, the how and why behind the symptoms you fixate on, the whole behind the healing, which cannot be found at the bottom of a bottle of pills.

But you do not speak this language. And so my sick sisterhood, whose bodies have been felled by mysterious illnesses, bear the arcane names of men long dead, signifying their suffering with no cure, no hope. They are no longer themselves.

Into their dry hungry mouths are dropped pills not answers.

Prescriptions and descriptions of symptoms – not cures or laws to halt the toxic corporate world that is allowed to carry on felling us like trees in the Amazon…

Each woman is an Amazon. But she does not know it. Instead she is treated. Separately. Her pile of notes, her bills growing higher. Each one believes the sickness is hers alone. Each is sent home, ignored, tolerated.

Alone. In the darkness.

Until one day Medicine Woman arises within her.

And there in the centre of her pain she finds her outrage, her strength, her persistence as she searches for answers. She finds the will to die to this world and the right to live a different life where she is honoured for the value of her soul, not the sweat of her brow. She finds the courage to ask brave questions. To heal when they say she cannot.

She begins to understand the messages her body is sending...

Things are not right. In here... out there.

She begins to remember there is magic in her: the power to heal, the power to transform.

You, dear sister, may be the last bastion of sanity in a culture gone mad. In a world so toxic it cannot function, so numb it cannot even cry out for help, so disconnected it cannot heal. Except through the cells of our bodies.

Our sisters are dying right now to tell you,

Enough suffering, it is time to heal.

MEDICINE QUESTIONS

Were you familiar with the term 'paradigm shift' before reading this book? How has your understanding developed or changed since reading this chapter?

Have you experienced a paradigm shift yourself in your lifetime? How did it happen? What did it feel like? Have you witnessed it happen on a larger scale before?

Can you create a graphic representation of the current paradigm?

What do you think comes next? How do you know this? Are you playing a part in this shift?

INITIATION

INVITATION

A major illness or injury is a rupture that invites you to rethink, to restart, to review what matters. It's a reminder that your time is finite and not to be wasted, and in breaking you from the past it offers the possibility of starting fresh. An illness is many kinds of rupture from which you have to stitch back a storyline of where you're heading and what it means.
Rebecca Solnit, *The Faraway Nearby*

Serious illnesses follow the stages and requirements of traditional initiation ceremonies – separation, submergence, metamorphosis and re-emergence.
Kat Duff, *The Alchemy of Illness*

Illness offers us an invitation. One that we may not have been expecting. Nor perhaps wished for. An invitation to initiation. Without an RSVP. We will be required to attend. There is no mistaking to whom the envelope was addressed. Its contents are life changing.

Normal is redefined. Consciousness recalibrated. Happily-ever-after has a question mark firmly placed after it.

Illness offers us an invitation that may feel like the end of the world. Like the lights being turned off. Like numb dread, screaming panic, searing pain. Where one moment is normal and the next your life is changed forever. Where your heart drops out of your body in terror and your mind spins off into outer space with the implications. Or perhaps it is a slow-building crescendo of shapeless hints and symptoms that have no form, no answer, only fuzziness and not-rightness.

Illness is an initiation into the worldly institutions of illness: the hospital routines, drug names and doses – as well as the incantations of illness. We order our days around them. Three times a day, take a pink one; half of the yellow, before dinner only, not after nine, no alcohol. When you take one step back, you can see the ritual is in many ways no different to magic.

That is the outer initiation. If you choose it. If you consent.

Illness offers another initiation, too, an inner initiation to the body – to feeling, releasing, healing what has been held in. It is a making public of what has been private, shining light on what has lain unseen. Sickness is a gift, wrapped up in the oddest, scariest, least obvious of wrappings: it brings us, if we will let it, back home to ourselves.

We can be guided by those who have walked that path before, or those who have been taught the signs and arts. But ultimately we walk this inner path alone. And there are no guarantees of success, nor even clarity of what this might look like. This is the inner initiation of the soul through the suffering of the body.

Illness initiates us, one way or the other. Or both.

It brings you to your knees, to rediscover sacred ground. Right here on your bathroom floor. Right here in your body.

Sickness is an existential striptease… it rips away the superficial, the window dressing, your costumes and masks, down to your naked emotions, naked bodies, your guts. It strips away your previous identities and roles and asks – *who are you really?*

It may be the first day of your life, the prime of youth or several decades in, when Medicine Woman calls you. Your name on her list. Her new initiate. She crept in whilst you were sleeping, when you overexerted, when you kissed him, or ate that, or lived there or pushed too hard just one time too many. She crept in and curled up in your cells, your heart, your brain, waiting to meet you. Longing to know you. Longing for you to know her, at last.

And what feels like the end is in fact a beginning, of a new road, an unknown path of pain and healing. She will show you how to slow down, she will run her fingers roughly through your life and help you sort the busyness from what matters. She will show you how to find

support... and who you really are, beyond your roles and expectations... and even more beyond the System the world has forced you
into. She will transport you into the timelessness of big pains and tiny
joys, initiate you into your strength, into your love, into your courage.
Into a world beyond your control.

She has sent me an invitation. I see yours too, tucked in your bag,
amongst all the receipts and bills, the pens and detritus of life.

Take it out. Shake off the crumbs, smooth out the creases.

It is time to step into the void and meet her.

$\bigcirc$

THE VOID

I don't know where I am.
I don't know who I am.
I don't know what will happen.

This is the void.
This is the darkness that must be known,
The terror of unbelonging, of death and dissolution.
The terror of the absence of self.
The hell of endless suffering.
You find yourself here, awake,
Hanging by a thread
Over the darkness you have run from all your life.
This is
Death.
Your carefully crafted persona
Lies in pieces,
Your body hangs on a meat hook,
Dripping.
Darkness.
Pain.
Fear.

Yet still you are here, precious one,
Still you are here.
You may get to the void through the numbing of medication.
You may get to it through despair or the deafening white noise of pain
or depression.
Disorientated in the darkness,
You have reached rock bottom
Yet still you are falling.
No light at the end of the tunnel.
Nowhere left to turn, no one left to trust.
Darkness everywhere.
This is the heroine's journey.
This is the initiation of the soul.
This is the path you will take, you must take.
This is the initiation of Medicine Woman.
Falling into the heart of paradox
Where black and white can no longer be seen.
Still you fall.
Perhaps letting go is not what you expected.
Perhaps the darkness is not to be feared.
Perhaps behind the pain lies something else.
Perhaps behind the fear is something different.
Perhaps you are not who you thought.
You are still here, precious one.
Open your eyes.
Breathe deep.
Let go.
Hold on.
Rest into the paradox of transformation.
Dare to trust the process.

MEDICINE WOMAN
– A LOST FEMININE ARCHETYPE OF HEALING

They called her witch because she knew how to heal herself.
Té V. Smith, *Here We Are, Reflections of a God Gone Mad*

When silence no longer serves you, when healing calls your name.
I will be waiting for you
Here in the shadows
To show you another way.

Who is Medicine Woman?

To me, Medicine Woman is an archetype, an energy force, the ancient soul of healing. To you she may be real: a goddess, a vision, a guide. She connects us to the wisdom of nature, to the primal electricity that has been tapped and held by cultures and their healers for millennia before man-made power turned on the lights. Medicine Woman is she who has walked this world and healed for a hundred thousand years before the gleam of steel and the coming of machines. She is the Feminine principle in healing that has been lost in our technocratic war on disease.

Medicine Woman is the teacher who cannot be seen with worldly eyes, the holder of the map to the mysterious road to healing. In one hand she holds honey – the golden elixir of life, sweetness and healing to stomach and soul, balm to the aching body. In the other she holds a bone knife – to cut away the old, the dead, the decayed. She knows that healing needs both. She teaches impermanence, surrender, the beauty and potential of endless transformation. She swipes away the ego, the shell, the identity and asks you to see what lies beneath. And beneath that too.

Medicine Woman's role is not to fix us so we can carry on, but to hold us as we transform. She is the guardian of our transition space, the womb within which we grow. She helps us to love what is, accept whatever this moment brings, whether we choose it or not. Hers is the presence of experience, the wisdom that has been carved canyon-deep through the suffering and love of all who have walked before us.

She is the inner midwife, shaman, grandmother, doula, the one who is with-woman. She sits by our side in the dark and holds space for the fullness of us to emerge.

Medicine Woman is she of the cycles. She who is poised between shedding and renewal, life and death. She who inhabits the crossroads, the space of decisions with unknowable consequences. She moves between the underworld and this world with ease. She of the bones, she of the soft flesh. She of compassion. She of unflinching tough love and tenderness.

She does not promise happily-ever-after but wisdom: that life is change, and that we will be changed by what we experience. That we will be marked by the pain we live through, the choices we make. Our experiences of suffering will shape us.

She is the one who rips the plaster off and shows us the magic and horror that lies below. The one who gifts us with scars and burns memories into our minds to remember her visit when she is gone. She tests us for weakness... and shows us that strength may not be what we have been taught. That our true strength lies in compassion, in our ability to weather adversity, to survive that which we think we cannot, and be humbled by that which we thought we could manage. She shows us again and again that we are not necessarily who we thought ourselves to be, that nothing is fixed, everything changes, and chaos lies just below the surface of what we think of as stability.

Medicine Woman is the great transformer, the spinner, the wheel turner, from life to death a thousand times we travel in our lifespan. She is able to stand in the face of death, and not back down. Death is not her master. She teaches us to take the pain, loss and grief and transform them, recycle them, transmute them into healing, into art, into compassion, into hope, into medicine, into pure love for ourselves and others. She is the queen of integration, teaching us how to weave together opposites, milling paradox and possibility. She teaches us to stop attaching to single outcomes, or to anything except the endless unfolding process of chaos and possibility.

Medicine Woman is she who remains when our consciousness shifts from its daily ways. She is there as we cross from waking to sleep, from pain to pleasure, from grief to acceptance. She stands as guardian, holding space for our return, offering her presence, holding the many threads of us in her wise hands. She bears witness as your soul reconnects with your body: the primal tear of being rejoined.

Medicine Woman is the Great Mother of your timeless self. She reacquaints you with your native magic, your ancient knowing, your wisdom beyond learning, your power to heal. She is your direct connection to the divine, the sacred, the life-force. She is the key to unlocking your wholeness, your healing. She speaks through metaphors, symbols, anomalies, miracles, coincidence and synchronicity. She speaks through touch and feeling. She is the principle behind healing that cannot be proven. She is the truth behind the illness and the cure. She is the everything between life and death that is felt but cannot be touched. She is the dimension that modern medicine is missing.

Medicine Woman has ancient roots, woven between the worlds, between body and soul, reality and other realms. Many cultures have their own understanding of her powers, and their own earthly lineages of her apprentices: medicine people with closely guarded rituals, skills in herbs, abilities to speak with spirits and lay on hands. They may be known as the shaman, the wise woman, the witch, the healer, the priestess, the midwife, the wyrd woman: all are embodiments of Medicine Woman.

She who works with the understanding of Medicine Woman, whatever her heritage or tradition, reclaims her own inner authority, reclaims her own direct connection to nature and the sacred, as she reclaims Feminine ways of healing and feeling.

The woman who has been touched by Medicine Woman learns how to step back, how to watch and listen. She is guided by her inner knowing. She is the midwife who knits through the hours before dawn, trusting the contractions that bring new life through. She is the therapist who reminds you how to breathe in the darkness of a panic attack. She is the nurse who wipes your brow in the dark fear of night, the mother who reminds you to eat your greens, who holds you as you sob. She who wraps a warm soft blanket around your shoulders when you shiver, who tells you to hold your nose and swallow the bitter medicine that will do you good. She who gets you to sit down and have a steaming cup of tea and listens as you unburden yourself, cradling its warmth between your hands. The wise one who knows that the goodness in your bones will pour out as you soak in a hot salt bath. Hers is the arm around your waist as you hobble, the hand on your elbow steering you gently when you are anxious and confused. Hers is the kiss on your cheek as gentle as a butterfly's wing as you drift to sleep after hours of hot, lonely tears in the middle of the night. Hers is the ear at the end of the emergency hotline, the fierce nurse who keeps uninvited visitors from your sick room, who plumps your pillow and firmly demands a second opinion. She is the one reminding you to take your pills each morning and whose hand you squeeze to the bone when the pain is too much to bear alone. She is the one who, when your fear becomes the size of the world, holds you gently but firmly and whispers: *you are safe, you are not your fear.* She is the one who steps back so that you can step forward. She is your courage, your permission, your sanctuary, your strength in the midst of suffering. She is your compassion for yourself and all around you. She is in your bones. You are she.

A medicine woman is a seer of patterns, a speaker of uncomfortable truths, a feeler of that which we have been taught not to feel, a namer, not only for herself but her community. Initiated by her illness she learns new ways of being: living in balance within herself, engaging with her energetic system on a more primal level. She learns the value and necessity of grief in order to fully release the old and embrace the new. She lives intimately the cycle of growth and decay. She learns to listen with her whole being – not just her outer eyes and ears, but her inner ones even more keenly. She uses her heightened sensitivity to feel beyond herself, into other realms and worlds, to gather information, to understand herself and the bigger picture. She begins to see beyond the veil. She becomes aware of the complexity of the environment within which she lives – the climate, seasons, other people's energy, her own, the impact of food, chemicals, nature and all other things on her body for good and ill.

When we allow integration, when we see beyond black and white, when we embrace complexity and paradox, then we become students of Medicine Woman. When we learn to embody her wisdom, to take an active role in healing ourselves… and the world… when we learn to transmute our pain into healing and share these gifts beyond ourselves, then we become the medicine women of our communities.

So I ask you, what if being sick was our medicine to a world gone wrong?

What if the years of suffering, silencing yourself, devaluing yourself, ignoring your needs, discrediting your truth, being poisoned, starved, overfed, overwhelmed, undervalued, trying to be what the world wanted, have brought you to this moment?

The opportunity to return to yourself.

You stand at the cross roads.

One way points down the recommended route of medical healing and cultural stigma. One points to continued denial. And the third lies in the shadows, the hidden arm of the finger-post leads to a path less travelled. Which to try, which to trust with your life?

There is something beneath your symptoms, beneath what our medical system can see that is broken, disconnected, mourning deeply. Something that may be dulled by your medication. Something.

In the midst of your madness, your fear and your pain you have found your way here in the darkness. To the heart of healing.

You have heeded the call of Medicine Woman.

The call of life herself.

This is your initiation.

If you step out of the life you had,

The life they told you that you must lead,

And step, with shaking faith, onto another path.

If you are prepared to step out of our sick culture for a moment

You will find yourself, at last, in the healing place.

You will discover the truth that has been hidden from you all along:

You are the medicine, woman.

MEDICINE QUESTIONS

Medicine Woman

Have you come across Medicine Woman before? If so, where? What did you previously know about her?

What resonance does Medicine Woman have for you? What mystery does she hold?

How do you understand her?

Do you have any women that you identify as medicine women within your community or culture? What have you learned from them?

How do you embody her? How have you resisted or rejected her in the past?

The Void

How are you at being in the darkness – literal and metaphorical? If this is new to you, I recommend my book, *Burning Woman*, which explores masculine and feminine darkness in great detail.

What memories and emotions does the darkness awaken in you?

How can you stay connected to your source, your wisdom within the darkness?

How can you stay connected to those around you?

How have you experienced the void before? What were you taught about it?

What will have to die? How much of you must go?

How can you let go? What has been your previous experience of letting go?

What can you hold on to?

What can you trust as you let go?

HEALING ARTS

Medicine Woman

Create an image of the archetype of Medicine Woman. What does she look like? What symbols represent her? What tools does she use? Paint her on the earth, draw her, collage or art journal her. Sculpt her from clay or papier mâché, needle-felt or knit her... what colour and form suits her best?

Where might you keep her so her presence is visible to you as you continue to read this book?

The Heroine's Journey

One of the scariest things about our descent – physical and emotional – into the void is the feeling of being lost, alone and without a map. Can you map the terrain of the void as you walk through it?

Can you paint or draw what the void looks like to you? What colour is it? What qualities does it have?

We are going to try to connect with the experience of the void visually. The first part is inspired by an exercise from Julie Gibbon's *Mandala Magic* course.

◯ Take several thick sheets of paper and gather a variety of art materials. You might want to try watercolour, soft pastels, oil pastels, acrylic paints, inks, charcoal from a store or from a fire you have lit yourself – perhaps even a ritual burning of something you want to be rid of... On each piece of paper use one of the selected media to create a large black circle. Stay fully connected to the feeling of being in the void as you do. Take as much time as you need to, allowing yourself to enjoy the sensations of creating this dark circle, the feeling of the materials in your fingers. Reflect on the different qualities that each of the materials bring to the look and feel of the void.

Reflect on the space around the void – do you want to leave it blank, use a different medium in the same or a different colour? What is the relationship between the void and what lies beyond it? Whereabouts are you right now? Are there any words you want to add in – around the outside or in the middle of the piece, any symbols or images? You could use ink, a pen or paint. Do you want them to show up or be in the same colour and medium as the void itself? How do you feel making this representation of the void? Do any new thoughts or feelings emerge for you as you do it? Journal about your feelings afterwards.

Ⓘ **The next exercise is for you if you are currently living in the void space: depressed, fearful or anxious.**

Brave heroine, you have travelled far to be here. Your courage is to be commended. I know that you have wandered the void space long-time and alone. The darkness here may have felt terrifying, but can you conceive of it as a gentler space, a womb space that can hold you as you transform. A sacred cocoon within which magic is happening unseen. Are you able to allow yourself to rest here, to stop your inner churning and struggle, and trust the process? Dare you trust that this agitation is not a sign of impending physical death, but an inner dying so that you can be reborn stronger?

If you feel you have done your time here but cannot find your way out, look around you with first your inner and then your outer eyes. What lifelines can you see? Is there a hand in the distance you can reach for? Perhaps the hand of a friend, family member, neighbour, pet or partner? You do not need to say anything, simply reach towards it in your mind's eye, with your energy body. Allow yourself to be energetically pulled gently out of this place by their love and care. Perhaps you can raise your voice to add to this energetic leaning – what do you need to say? *Help… help me…. I'm stuck… I'm scared…* Say it quietly under your breath right now. Then a bit louder. Who do you want to hear this? A friend, family member, neighbour, partner, doctor, counsellor, your god or goddess, perhaps a kind anonymous human at the end of a phone line who knows how to listen?

Can you try to draw a map of where you are right now or write a description of what the place you are in feels like and looks like? Where can you leave it or who can you give it to, so that the people who care about you can find you?

① **The next exercise must not be done alone if you are currently living in the void space, extremely depressed, fearful or anxious. Instead explore your responses to the questions with a trusted friend or counsellor.**

Make sure you are in a safe, quiet and comfortable physical space where you will not be disturbed for at least half an hour, preferably somewhere that is not too bright. Allow yourself to hold onto something tangible – perhaps a pebble or stick in your hand to root you back here in your earthly body. Know that at all times you can simply squeeze this object and open your eyes and you will be safe and back in the world. In this exercise you are going to take an inner journey of reflection into the void and the Heroine's journey. If you are unsure of what I mean by the Heroine's journey you might want to read or listen to the myth of Persephone, Psyche or Inanna first.

Take some time to look at your favourite void image that you created. Let your vision soften, and perhaps close your eyes. Allow yourself to take an imaginary journey into the void, and down into the darkness of the Underworld. Have you passed this way before? If so, what wisdom do you remember for this journey? What are the major landmarks? Are there lakes, rivers, mountains, trees, valleys, gates or portals? What might they be called? Can you mentally create a map of the Underworld that you can later draw or write out for yourself or others who follow after?

What does the Heroine who is passing this way look like? Is she you as you are now, you from a different time in your life, a mythical version of you, or someone else entirely? What does she carry? Does she have any weapons, tools or skills that help her here? What questions would you like to ask her about this place and the purpose of your visit here?

Are there any magical allies or guides to this realm that you can summon up? What form do they take? Are they human, superhuman, animal, elemental or landscape features? How do they communicate? What lessons do they have to teach you about your fear, your illness, your current life situation or relationships?

Look around you, perhaps ask the Heroine or allies what you can bring back into the daily world with you to remind you of your time here and the lessons learned. Take a few more moments here, and then squeeze your hand around the pebble, take a deep breath into your belly and open your eyes. Allow yourself to stay fully with your body as you acclimatise to being back in the everyday.

You may want to take a few minutes to journal or sketch your experiences. Over the coming days take time to find or craft an object, image or symbol that represents this Underworld journey and wear it, keep it on an altar space, in your purse or on a windowsill to remind you of what you have learned.

You may want to discuss this sacred Heroine's journey to the Underworld with a trusted friend, counsellor or women's circle, to share what you have learned, and receive additional insight from your trusted worldly allies. Be sure to pay extra attention to your dreams for the next few nights and to messengers and synchronicities in the everyday world.

THE ART OF HEALING

THE SOUL OF HEALING

You have travelled too fast over false ground;
Now your soul has come, to take you back.
John O'Donohue,
from 'For One Who is Exhausted', *Benedictus*

When the land is taken by the patriarchy where can we go to heal?
Inwards, inwards.
Guided by the presence of Medicine Woman,
Into a place
Where the soul of healing resides,
Where the old can be shed, removed, laid to rest and
New possibility can be visioned, stepped into, rooted deep.
Let us reclaim this space,
It is time to dance our healing and paint it in bright colours.

The word *healing*, meaning "to restore sound health", shares its roots with the term 'wholeness'. So, if sickness is considered the disintegration of the bodymind's healthy functioning, healing is what helps us put the pieces back together.

We know the outer terrain of physical medicine. It is well lit, well signposted and well-travelled in our culture. If you break your leg Western medicine knows how to mend your bones and retrain your weakened muscles. It knows the pathways of nerves to avoid during surgery, the correct levels of anaesthetic and the best practice for avoiding sepsis.

But once we move from healing tendons and bones and into the less tangible but no less real terrain of the psyche or soul: what illness or injury means to us, how it affects our sense of identity and self-esteem, into the meaning of pain and how to survive it, how to navigate the darkness of loss and suffering, how our minds impact our healing process, Western medicine gets lost, still trying to approach with tablets and scalpels things which cannot be seen, touched or tested.

Healing and curing are not synonymous,[111] though Western medicine tries to pretend they are. Where the aim of curing is the end of symptoms – the disappearance of cancer or the replacement of a diseased organ – healing is a coming into balance both within ourselves and with the world around us. We can in fact be healed but not cured, and cured but not healed. So, for example, an operation may be deemed successful because it has cured the physical problem, but the emotional and spiritual trauma that may have been caused in the process of 'curing' are often minimised and overlooked, yet can be as debilitating as the original injury. Whereas someone may choose not to take any more medication and therefore die from what ails them, but in making peace with themselves and their loved ones in their final days, they may find deep healing, even though they are not cured.

What healing actually *is* and *where* it comes from is still a contentious issue, depending on our beliefs. For some the answer might be our cells, for others it might be God or the body's innate intelligence. I found the following explanation a great way of stripping away these differences of belief, to allow us to see what might be needed for healing and how we might access it:

At the most fundamental level, everything is energy. Energy is simply potential until different patterns arise within that energy. Patterns are like the blueprint of physical existence. Because everything is a pattern, all forms of illness are also specific patterns. Therefore, the first layer to understand about healing is that to heal is to change a pattern. It is the opposite of repetition and redundancy.

When something is unhealed, it is exhibiting a pattern that we don't like. It is in a state that is unwanted. We can greatly simplify healing in that it is a change of a pattern that is unwanted into a pattern that is wanted. This usually entails changing it into the opposite pattern.

[…] To heal anything, we must 'experience the opposite'. We must experience what is wanted, instead of what is unwanted.

If our leg is broken, to change that pattern of broken into its opposite is to put together/mend.

If we feel demeaned, to heal is to feel valued.

If we are abused, to heal is to be treated lovingly.

If we feel powerless, to heal is to feel empowered.[112]

At its most basic, healing can be understood as the ultimate creative act: that of alchemy or magic. It is the turning of one state into another: the negative into the positive, the darkness and shadow into gold – by engaging medicines, the life-force, our conscious and unconscious mind, as well as harnessing the powers that lie within and beyond us.

Within our current paradigm, sickness is discounted as a purely bad thing because it disables the physical body and the brain. The gifts and insights that come with it are not considered relevant. And so, when it comes to the inner journey of healing we are left to our own devices. We do everything we can to avoid it, rather than respect the process of illness and healing and the tremendous positive transformations it can bring both to an individual and a community.

When our focus is solely on functionality, on the physical, then the harder to define, yet no less important other realms of our humanity can be completely overlooked as superfluous, in the rush to shrug off the disability of sickness and get back to normal. When the only reality our culture acknowledges is the one we can see and touch – not the intangible energy of thought, feeling, history, lineage, ancestors, archetypes, meaning, identity and belief, we miss what makes us human. The unseen part of ourselves, the soul, the consciousness which pours through us, is completely ignored.

When we do acknowledge the unseen aspects of healing in the West, it tends to be either through the framework of religion or through the pervasive lens of commercialised New Age spiritual understanding. The first mistake we often make is the one I shared at the beginning of the book, the quick-fix recommended to us by so many self-help books, motivational speakers and evangelists of all stripes: trying to positively think ourselves out of sickness. But the more entrenched we become in our minds and the more we try to block, force, or deny the reality of the body, the more cut off we become from our embodied experience, the less able we are to respond to what our bodies actually need to heal: the expression and elimination of what is sickening them, and building up what they are deficient in.

So, let me be clear that whilst the focus of this section is on the soul of healing, I am not calling for us to walk away from using logic, testing, research or otherwise applying our mental faculties to healing our bodies. But rather to acknowledge that our physical body is only a *part* of us. And to heal the whole of us, we cannot apply the skills and the logic of just one part. And this is what has happened with the attempted Western rationalisation of medicine: the logical left brain has dominated other ways of knowing, and the body's innate intelligence. The science of medicine has colonised and dominated the art of healing. But both art and science are both desperately needed now as we enter into the new territory our species finds itself in. We need ancient wisdoms *and* modern technology and theories. We need body, mind and soul. We need to bring our whole selves to healing.

DECOLONISING SOUL

We had a lot of trouble with Western mental health workers who came here immediately after the genocide. They came and their practice did not involve being outside in the sun where you begin to feel better, there was no music or drumming to get your blood flowing again, there was no sense that everyone had taken the day off so that the entire community could come together to try to lift you up and bring you back to joy, there was no acknowledgement of the depression as something invasive and external that could actually be cast out again. Instead they would take people one at a time into these dingy little rooms and have them sit around for an hour or so and talk about bad things that had happened to them. We had to ask them to leave.
A Rwandan talking to a Western writer, Andrew Solomon.

Despite illness being a factor common to every human across cultures and throughout time, when we find ourselves in the place of sickness in the West, we find ourselves on the very edge of our cultural narrative: it makes us deeply uncomfortable. Sickness does not fit with who we see ourselves as being. And our medical system reinforces this.

When we first get sick, we try to grasp for the familiar: seeking help from known and trusted places. But if these fail us or lose our trust, we begin to look elsewhere.

In this globalised world we have the option of reaching out beyond the cultural practices of Western medicine, to a whole host of alternatives: an option that so many of our ancestors did not have. These alternatives often seem more soulful, exotic and inviting than the prosaic reality of an overcrowded family doctor's waiting room, or a tablet with unknown side effects.

But we tend to do this within the capitalist paradigm we have been raised, believing, as our forefathers taught us, that everything has a price, that everything is ours for the taking.

I, like so many white women, find myself like a hungry ghost, with a soul that has been cut off from its native sources of healing and a bodymind that has been conditioned from birth within capitalist patriarchy. I both belong to this culture by the colour of my skin, my middle-class roots, my heterosexual family set-up, the culture in my cells, the tongue I speak, the history I share – and I do not by dint of my unorthodox family, my lack of mainstream religion, my neurotype, my gender and my mental health issues.

My own heritage is predominantly Celtic, the mystical outsiders to the Anglo-Saxon world. On both sides I am Irish, Welsh, Scottish, with large dashes of English and Polish thrown in for good measure. I have been raised in the cradle of European patriarchy by conscientious objectors, religiously non-conformist, bohemian self-employed creatives.

There are medicine women in the roots of my culture, in our mythology, but they have been lost to me, just as they have been lost to most of us inhabitants of the dominant modern cultures. Warmongers, politicians and priests systematically destroyed so much of our indigenous culture and healing at home to cement their own dominance, before moving on to colonise the globe, destroying the indigenous spiritual and healing cultures of every place they landed. Healing in traditional ways was outlawed, punished, ridiculed, the culture and soul of each people was consciously broken, just as their bodies and minds were sickened, forcibly replaced by patriarchal law, religion, education and medicine, in the supposed desire to enlighten and save.

And so we find ourselves here, in the fast-paced modern world, orphaned from our motherland whilst living in the fatherland. In a culture that is ours, but that does not feel like ours. We find ourselves trying to become the medicine women we need, that our culture needs, with few or no elders to initiate us. We have few indigenous practices to inherit and so find ourselves in the uncomfortable privileged position of trying to borrow or learn from the cultures that our forefathers tried to destroy. And trying to mend a broken inner connection without much guidance and few reference points, within a birth culture that openly mocks and criticises us.

In doing so we often mistake witnessing the vibrant, living soul of others for our own. In the parched thirst we have for soul, we do not realise that the soul we are coveting is not ours to take. It cannot make us better, because it is not ours. We can learn from careful observation the practices that assist the cultivation of soul, but we cannot buy or steal it. We can only take this journey of soul reclamation ourselves, our privilege cannot buy us a quick pass to happily-ever-after.

There is an ever-present danger, in our desperation to heal, in our aversion to pain, that we look for short cuts. That we appropriate things from the cultures of others, which in our coloniser mentality we can do so easily, taking practices piecemeal, disregarding their roots, whilst still passively or actively contributing to the destruction of the culture they came from.

We cannot shy away from this. It is not about judgement or blame, but real seeing, real acknowledgement of the pain that our ancestors have caused in others, that we still cause in others, that we have numbed ourselves to. Just as we have numbed the pain in ourselves. It is one and the same. We can only heal when we can see this, when we can feel the pain as our own, when we do not isolate ourselves from it, when we do not allow ourselves to disconnect from the suffering of others.

We must understand and acknowledge the ways we have internalised patriarchal values unknowingly: for we are not just victims of it. As much as it pains us to admit it, we are also the perpetrators of this sick culture. But we are no longer powerless. We are both the sickness and the potential for healing.

LEARNING TO LISTEN

Though her soul requires seeing, the culture around her requires
sightlessness. Though her soul wishes to speak its truth,
she is pressured to be silent.
Clarissa Pinkola Estés, Women Who Run With the Wolves

People start to heal the moment they feel heard.
Cheryl Richardson

If a woman's body is a book, it is written in the Feminine, our native tongue. Our bodies speak eloquently. And yet, we have been taught that because they do not speak English, they are dumb. *Speak the dominant language or die* is the approach of colonialism. We have internalised this directive. And so we have relied on the appointed translators of the body – the medical men – to interpret our bodies and relay the information back to us in their antiquated Greek terms. Where there are no equivalencies in terms of language or even concept, whole areas of female experience have been left blank and unspoken... and therefore also untreated.

The stories that sickness holds, the transformation it contains, the wisdom that we women have carried across time written on our bodies in the form of our illnesses and suffering, have often been the only way our souls have had of communicating directly with us. We have been told to ignore their realities so often, to silence our inner knowing, scorn our intuition, abandon our creativity, forget the past, cut off from our own connection to the mystery, deny our innate healing powers and defer to the experts so frequently that we no longer understand ourselves.

....

I have learned to see my health challenges as a much wiser teacher than
my conscious, ego-driven self. I used to feel such a victim, and so angry
that I'd been dealt such a rubbish hand.
But then I went through slow, incredibly painful annihilation and
through that process I simultaneously and completely broke down all the
preconceptions I had about health and wellbeing. I discovered miracu-

lous extra, abundant resources when my physical core had reached the brink of extinction. I tuned into the incredible power of the breath and utilised my practice every waking hour, experimenting with different techniques as I needed. To stay on top of the intense pain, discomfort, emotional trauma and chronic insomnia, I quickly learned to trust my intuition and follow those internal nudges – even when it would have been far easier to flip out. And gradually – as I began to see the painfully slow, totally non-linear healing take place in my body – something very new birthed in me: my spirituality. For the first time in my life, I surrendered myself to the universe and discovered with awe just how big, how connected and how supportive it truly is.

In short, I learned that I was suppressing myself in almost every layer of my being, and that resulted in my various chronic conditions.

*I'm now a passionate believer that healing is simply about full expression – not just creatively or cognitively, but in every one of your five energy bodies (body-breath-mind-power-spirit). If any one or more of these is currently being suppressed or denied in any way, the likelihood is you are feeling broken or less than. And there's good reason for that, because these five bodies are your ecosystem! When one breaks down the rest have to work much harder in order to keep **you** in some kind of balance.*

ZOË

Often the predominant feeling when we are ill is one of a deep alienation from our self. A belief that the body is failing us and that all that we know ourselves to be is crumbling. We lose trust in ourselves, in our bodies, in our abilities. In ensouling our bodies once more, we reclaim that which we have never lost but simply lost sight of. We remember our value beyond our economic contribution, social status, appearance and achievements – we remember the greater self that lies beyond all this, which has the right to exist and does not need to earn its place.

We remember that we, that all life, has inherent value, meaning and intelligence.

REMEMBERING WHAT MATTERS

I had tried medication and psychiatrists and resting and supplements and ignoring it. I was lying on the floor as panic attack after panic attack rolled through my body as I attempted to dress myself.

"None of it's working," my husband said, "we need to try something different."

I needed to remember what mattered.

Re-member, as in to take back into my body what mattered. To re-connect with the magic of life beyond the realms of my broken body and shattered mind.

My breathing settled. We waited there together in the doorway. Waited for the answer.

I told him I needed to do something my brain could handle, that my nervous system could manage without panic. Something that felt good and safe and healing.

He asked me what that would look like. I thought a moment, and then told him I needed to organise the spice drawer. This was one part cleaning (which I normally avoid like the plague), three parts organising which soothes my brain and five parts the chance to sift through spices with my fingers, to have the excuse to touch and smell them.

I needed to paint with my fingers, with no ambition other than to touch colours. I needed to plant seeds in the earth and watch them grow. I needed to stand on the seashore again. But I couldn't get there alone.

He drove me to the beach with our older daughter. We stood on the shore and talked. And played on the sand. And picked up pebbles. And laughed at silly things. And I felt alive. For the first time in weeks I was part of the world, not looking in on a place I was locked out of.

We went home. I made soup and brownies. And ate them. And felt alive. After months force-feeding myself or binging when I could eat.

And then we sat and watched the birds from our kitchen window. Rather than endless boxed sets on Netflix. We set a timer for ten minutes. In ten minutes we saw two birds at our feeder. But just watching them with a purpose felt good. Good to be connected to something outside of my own bodymind.

So I went outside and set that timer for ten more minutes and sat in a damp garden chair in the chill sunshine of a late January morning under the bare bones of the cherry tree and watched and listened for the birds. Ten minutes turned into twenty, the timer put aside. I could barely feel my fingers. But I was alive. Remembering just how beautifully small and insignificant I was. My pain seemed more manageable when accompanied by the robin's sweet song. My existence, for the first time in weeks was no longer negotiable, it just was, as much as the sunbeams filtering through the bare branches.

HEALING IS FEELING

Only that which is deeply felt can change us. Rational arguments alone cannot penetrate the layers of fear and conditioning that compromise our crippling belief systems.
Marilyn Ferguson, *The Aquarian Conspiracy*

Genuine feelings cannot be produced, nor can they be eradicated. We can only repress them, delude ourselves, and deceive our bodies. The body sticks to the facts.
Alice Miller, *The Drama of the Gifted Child*

We have been taught again. And again. And again. To override our feeling selves with our minds. This is the first lesson of patriarchy, taught from birth: *Do. Not. Feel.*

Some of us literally cannot feel what is going on in our bodies, we have trained ourselves so successfully to numb ourselves and deny the importance of them.

Some of us may not be able to identify *what* the sensations and emotions we have are – this is called alexithymia.

Some of us have never been taught the language to describe the feelings we have inside.

Some of us have learned that to give expression – verbal or otherwise – to our feelings is dangerous, because of the reactions of others around us, or our own intense feelings.

Some of us do not have anyone we feel safe to share our feelings with.

Most of us do not have a full bag of effective tools and techniques to explore and express our inner feelings.

Sickness is a crash course in body literacy. In seeing, listening to and acknowledging so many parts of our bodies, our pasts, our selves that we have been more comfortable ignoring: parts that our culture and family have raised us to ignore, would prefer us to ignore. It is a picking apart of the white noise that has shaped us.

Sickness brings us uncomfortably back to ourselves, the fullness of ourselves: the dark as well as the light. It reacquaints us with our pain, fear, anger, grief, sadness, frustration, despair, powerlessness. Our trauma. Our loss. The vulnerability we have spent a lifetime trying to deny. All those feelings that we tend to naturally push away. All those states of being that our culture encourages us to ignore. Silence. Or cover with a smile. It also often connects us with states of being that are normally shut off to us in our daily lives: the far reaches of consciousness that few travel in our culture.

··

As part of my condition is congenital, I was in effect 'born this way' and despite not being fully diagnosed until the age of forty, I do in some way feel vindicated that the pain I suffered as a child, and throughout adulthood, was not merely a figment of my imagination, the outcome of overly fussy parenting (nothing could be further from the truth!) or a symptom of psychological illness or female over-sensitivity or emotionality as is so often the accusation levelled by doctors who are unable to work out the cause of pain. I was taught not to trust the signals (pain) my body was sending me to alert me to the fact that something was wrong. I was taught to second-guess and doubt my instincts about my own body.

HELEN

··

Our culture has been based on suppression. The suppression of Nature. The suppression of the Feminine. The suppression of the individual's own nature: our libidos, creative expression, direct connection to spirit and emotional feelings. Much of our physical pain is the more acceptable expression of this submerged psychological pain: the suppressed self fighting to be free.

And so now here we are, those of us whose minds were a little broken by trauma, whose bodies were a little broken by illness, whose spirits have been a little broken by abuses along the way, whose systems have been infected and made toxic. And we cannot sustain the suppression any longer. Our bodies are breaking the code of silence, they are starting to express this in aches and pains and rashes and tiredness. And when they do we are told to repress, quickly, once more.

But we find this time that we cannot.

We must not.

Our bodies are singing. Let us listen before they fall forever silent.

Now is our time to take a stand. We are at last consciously experiencing the wholesale sacrifice of the Feminine on the altar of patriarchal capitalism. We are experiencing the pain of this trauma in our bodyminds that has been unconscious for so long. The Feminine is awakening within us as individuals and a species, to take one last stand for life, to stop our culture sleepwalking into death.

Medicine Woman is awakening within us. She is calling us to heal our systems, to heal the System.

Before it is too late.

Throughout our lives we have been told time and again that we shouldn't have these feelings in our bodies, shouldn't feel them if we do. We certainly shouldn't express them. We are told it is these feelings that are wrong. We are told we are bad for feeling this way. And so we feel bad. All the time. Physically. Emotionally. We tell ourselves that we are wrong for feeling the way we know we shouldn't.

But still we feel this way. And so we keep very quiet about this. We know we shouldn't be experiencing reality the way we are, and so conclude that there is something wrong with us.

But it is not us. It is only our silence and shame that keep us from seeing how *human*, how real, how *normal* our feelings are. And then we realise, there is nothing *wrong* with us for feeling this way, nothing wrong with feeling: it is simply that the open expression of inner feeling is the enemy of the patriarchy. Because it disrupts their projections of superficial perfection, and lets the chaotic, creative inner darkness leak through.

*I really went through a deep process of taking ownership of what was
happening to me, because it helped me make sense of it – discovering
how this illness was the result of different events in my life and their
accumulation: from nearly dying in the womb and the physiological
scars it left inside my body, as well as the effects of the drugs my mother
was put on; the depletion and exhaustion caused by pregnancy, breastfeeding, and how much pressure I put myself under to be a wonderful
mother; the crisis of identity created by sudden and unexpected motherhood, and the subsequent struggle to integrate pre-motherhood-me with
mother-me; to a lot of transformational work that I had done prior
to getting sick; as well as a lot of dental work (and subsequently the
discovery that I was highly allergic to the anaesthetic used).*
*I understand disease as an imbalance of health; I saw the disruption in
my internal ecology that had allowed infection and immune disfunction
to set in, I understood how much of a teaching, and indeed of a near-
shamanic process, this all was.*
*And then after over two years of this process, after a healing session,
enormous anger welled up inside me... And I realized I had been so
focused on taking responsibility for all of this, I had never allowed myself
to get angry. Angry that it happened to me! Destroyed life as I knew it!
Damaged my children's childhood, my love relationship, my friendships!
That it was so fucking unfair, and I was allowed to rebel, and say NO!
To indeed see those bacteria that were eating me inside as invaders, even
if my understanding of health was much broader and I knew there were
so many other layers of understanding, but I was allowed also to see them
as foreign invaders, and kick them out of my body, because it was **mine**.*
In other words, big boundary issues came to light.
*That was a turning point in my getting better, as I was then ready to do
anything it took.*

FLORENCE

Sickness can be seen as a thawing of the personal permafrost due to
climate change: what has lain hidden beneath – the fossils and meth-
ane and rotten matter – all come to the surface together. The result
can be totally overwhelming and disabling: an assault on all our bodily

systems, a clash and fusing together of the deep past and the present in an uncomfortable mess.

When we embark on deep healing, rather than superficial curing, we have to release the pain which once was emotional but has hardened into physical suffering. We do this by learning to tap into the old parts of ourselves, the primal parts that we have silenced and ignored. We learn to take responsibility for ourselves, this is very different to taking the *blame* for them.

As women's doctor Christiane Northrup astutely observes: "Feeling that we are to blame for our illnesses simply reconstellates the woundings of our childhood and is exactly the opposite of healing. Feeling we are to blame keeps us stuck and unable to move forward in our healing. The part of us that 'creates an illness' is *not* the part of us that feels the pain of the illness. It is not a conscious part of us, but it can be affected by our consciousness once we put our healing process to work."

It is no surprise that those of us who have the most hidden trauma, tend to see the greatest impact on our health in mid-life. The work on Adverse Childhood Experiences and trauma is showing what as a culture we have been in denial about: that psychological trauma creates physical damage. Repressed emotional experiences can compromise our immune systems years later. In the words of Bessel van der Kolk, "the body keeps the score."[114] The physical body is not, and never has been, isolated from the psyche: they are interwoven at all levels. And they are communicating with us always. But often we do not want to hear what they have to say. The less we listen, the louder they have to scream to be heard.

OUR HEALING IS CONNECTED

The anger that I feel is lashed out at you in supermarket checkout queues and airports and rush hour traffic.

The grief I feel eats away at my organs, which costs your taxes to heal.

The powerlessness I feel is enacted upon your body in terrorist attacks.

The ambulance I need is driven by your mother, the nurse I need is your brother.

The medicines I need are harvested by your cousin, dispensed by your neighbour, legislated against by her friend.

The medicines I take I share with you, with the fish and the seabirds, the algae and the whales.

The stress I feel is embodied by every person my life touches.

The healing I receive is also.

RE-MEMBERING SAFETY

Trauma is not what happens to us but what we hold inside in absence of empathetic witnesses.
Peter Levine

The truth about our childhood is stored up in our body, and although we can repress it, we can never alter it. Our intellect can be deceived, our feelings manipulated and our body tricked with medication. But someday our body will present its bill, for it is as incorruptible as a child, who, still whole in spirit, will accept no compromises or excuses, and it will not stop tormenting us until we stop evading the truth.
Alice Miller, *The Drama of the Gifted Child*

For those of us who are chronically stressed, eternally endangered, whose souls are exiled outside our unsafe-feeling bodies, we need to find a key to the door, a way back into our bodies. A way to feel safe. A way to stay here. A way to be able to feel, see and speak again. A way to re-connect body, mind and soul.

We need to find a way, at last, for our bodies to become our most trusted allies, our most precious homes. If the feeling of a safe home or trusted ally was not rooted in our bodies in early childhood, we need to excavate to the very foundations of our beings.

At the heart of healing for me, for most of us, has been re-membering safety in my body, in my mind, in this culture. Learning to feel safe in them again. Replacing trauma with safety.

Finding a trusted ally, a safe space where we can learn, little by little to feel safe in our bodies, safe with another, and eventually to come home to the world, tends to be the key. Finding safe hands to hold you as you heal and rebirth. Finding a soul community, a gentle and wise counsellor, a gifted intuitive body worker, a medicine man or woman whose healing tools work for you.

And when we find a way that we can re-member our primal safety we can at last re-connect with the life-force that has been constricted by our fear, and that holds our healing.

LETTING GO

Sometimes, madness seems like the only possible response to the insanity of the civilised world; sometimes, holding ourselves together is not an option, and the only way forwards is to allow ourselves to fall apart.
Sharon Blackie, *If Women Rose Rooted*

*The question is not: Will you die? The question is which **you** needs to die off so that the new self can live and thrive in a new loving world?*
Sue in Eve Ensler's *In the Body of the World*

On some level we resist healing because we are aware that the journey of healing usually has a high price. It tends to require letting a part of yourself, your psyche, your creation myth, your stories, a familiar archetype go. It may also entail the loss of a part of your physical body, a job or a relationship: letting go of the certainty you had and the normality you could feel safe in.

Healing requires that we find our way through the layers of the mind activated by sickness: the fear, the feeling of victimhood and emotional trauma it activates, and the stories we tell ourselves about our pain and suffering. When we can move through these, what we discover is that illness is a time of massive change – of simultaneous death and growth. Whether or not our bodies are *actually* dying during our illness, our minds believe that they too are dying.

In order to be able to fully heal we need two things. We have to be prepared to die. And we have to be fully prepared to live. To live more fully, differently, more vibrantly than we ever have before. To seize hold of life in one hand and death in the other and dedicate ourselves wholeheartedly to both. To die to our old bodies, our previous conceptions of self. We know that we are uncomfortable with death. But we may find we are also uncomfortable with life.

The transformation of the psyche in illness, whilst it requires a death, is actually more akin to the shedding of a shell. Think of a hermit crab, its soft body cannot protect itself from predators, and so it picks up a discarded shell and uses it as its home and refuge. But eventually the crab outgrows its shell and must shed it. This is the inner transformation of illness. Rather than a diminishment of self, which is what we first experience it as in the death stage, it is actually a time for growth, for finding a new shell that is big enough to contain and protect our expanded self. But, at the time of shedding, when we are running naked along the sand with the gulls wheeling above, eyeing our vulnerable soft bodies, we know just how dangerous this process is and we fear our impending death.

Healing requires that we become actively engaged with the physical and mental processes of death, birth, transformation and living – consciously engaging with and influencing processes, which are usually unseen and unconscious. For those of us who have been stacking up traumas, who have not had the skills or knowledge or time and space or support to deal with the pain, anger or grief as they came up previously, the learning curve is stepper and harder. And it's happening in the midst of our sickness.

Healing requires a letting go of many of the old stories and identities that we used to understand ourselves through, that we used to protect ourselves with, that we used to contain our denial: the Good Girl who was approved of by the patriarchy, the Victim, the patient, the saviour, the martyr, the hard worker, the perfect woman. It requires much grieving, far more than we or our culture are comfortable with, before we can begin to accept and embrace the new identities, new abilities, new limitations that we may not ever have chosen, but which have become our new reality anyway. This can be really scary. But my experience of this has been: when you do this, when you accept yourself as you are, when you communicate this reality honestly to those around you rather than hiding and pretending, life becomes easier, as you are no longer expending vast amounts of energy trying to sustain an illusion. You are met in your own reality.

[Being ill] taught me to let go and trust; sometimes that was all I could do. Fighting is a loss of energy, and when you've little of it to begin with, you've got to conserve it. And sometimes, for example if I was scared, I found I had no choice but to trust what was happening in my body and stop second-guessing everything. I had the experience of being very ill for my own growth and transformation, and to help others do the same – to learn from illnesses and become a stronger, different person on the other side. I think this never finishes, I think I will always still have more to learn.

CIARA

As well as a psychic death, illness brings us closer to the reality of our own physical death and our extreme physical vulnerability and lack of control over how and when this life ends. This may bring up the ghosts of those we have loved and lost to similar illnesses, the suffering that we saw them endure, the realisation that we will not be the parent we had hoped, the partner or friend we long to be. We may not be able to achieve what we wanted in the professional or creative world. We may mourn the lives we once had, the people we once were, the things we will never do, the places we will never go, the folks we will never see again.

We find ourselves stuck in limbo, not knowing how long we have left, what the quality of that life will be or if it will be bearable. We find ourselves alternately longing for the sweet release of death, the end of suffering and then clinging to life with every fibre of our being. Again and again we learn to die. Again and again we have to learn to live.

This, I know myself, and from talking to other women, is one of the most challenging aspects of illness. We are taught by our culture to get back to normal, to fight illness, to fight for recovery. The flipside is, for most of us at some point, we will need to surrender a part of our cherished bodies or abilities to illness. We will need to lay down things we love, or find new ways to do them. We will need to die to ourselves and those we love as the person we once were. And we will need to dare to enter the void to discover who we really are beneath these discarded shells of ourselves.

But in order to stop, or even slow down, we need to call in every resource we have – from friends and family, any savings and favours, any benefit payments and barters – to let up the pressure on our bodyminds. We need to break the unspoken female code of martyrdom. We have to figure out what we can drop. What pressures are self-imposed. What responsibilities can be shared. What standards can be lowered. What we can say no to today. What we can leave until tomorrow. What doesn't need to be done at all. What can be done in a simpler way.

Stopping is scary. It means everything we have been running away from catches up to us – our debts, responsibilities, fears, traumas, loneliness... But it also means that there is space and time for the good stuff to reach us too: the inner and outer supports and healing, more of our own energy, possibilities that we have been running blind past.

It is our choice. For now. We slow down. We stop now. Or our bodyminds stop us when we're suffering even more.

We get this choice multiple times a day. Each day.
Until the choice is taken out of our hands.
And major sickness or death stop us more permanently.
Reaching out for healing requires that we let go of fear
Of rejection for not living up to expectations.
We learn to fall from certainty into the arms of possibility.
We shed a skin. It feels like the end.
But it is just the end of what was.
The end of living a lie.
The skin falls.
Life continues. Snaking away. Ever onwards.

THE FIRST STEP TO HEALING

Pain travels through families until someone is ready to feel it.
Stephi Wagner

Your pain is the breaking of the shell that encloses your understanding.
Khalil Gibran

So how do you start the process of healing? What if I told you that has already started, my love. Your body and soul are embodying it right now. The only thing you need do is to let the process unfold.

Stop. Rest. As much as you can. Make space and time for yourself. And begin to listen. Deeply. Be fully present in your body and ask honestly:

What am I feeling right now?

Don't try to change it, or deny it, or explain it. Simply feel it. The hot, the cool, the anger, the trembling, the rushing of blood, the buzz and fizz, the numbness, the fear, the aching or stinging.

What am I feeling right now?

Descend further. Into the place between physical and emotional pain, into the place where there is no separation. Listen to the old stories that are emerging. Listen as they beg to be heard. Write them out, speak them, move them out, cry them out, breathe them out…

What am I feeling right now?

And begin, perhaps for the first time, to really feel your own reality, beyond cliché and words. Not what you should or shouldn't be feeling. Not what is acceptable or explicable, but what is true for you right now.

What am I feeling right now?

You may hear the voices you have tried to silence. The stories you have tried to erase. The visions you have tried to ignore. The feelings you have tried to numb. The fear, the fear, the fear, the habitual fear. They reach a crescendo as you prepare to run and hide from them once more. But what if you stayed with them right now, and watched them carefully, curiously? What if you were to wait with them and see what lies on the other side of fear? What if instead of resisting, fighting, hardening against the pain you were to soften towards it? Allow it to flow into the rest of your body, allow the energy it contains to dissipate and integrate into the rest of you.

When we drop the defenses we usually use to hold back the tide of feeling, in that moment we are forced to slow down to the pace of the body rather than race to the pace of the mind. When we can allow the feeling to exist, without attaching extra thoughts and stories to it, we begin once again to live at the pace of the breath, to trust what is unfolding, rather than the script we usually follow. Rather than trying to retreat further and further from the body into the mind or numbness, can we dare to move the other way, back into the body?

Often all we can manage is just this breath. But it is all we need to manage. Just this breath. And then the next. Just that. And as we focus on the breath, focus on travelling through this very moment rather than resisting it, we begin to notice that somewhere, somehow, something starts to shift, without our doing anything. The process is partnering us.

I am not my fear.

I am not my pain.

And when in time, the intensity has fallen away, when in time we can pull back from the solipsism of this moment, we can see the crystalline complexity of the process, the thousands of threads that have woven together to make it, the hundreds of shifts that have happened because of it. We can see the beauty of the world beyond us, the love and care that have been shown to us. We can pause and give thanks for small acts of kindness and realise that these are greater than the pain. In the moment of our suffering, the fear and the pain blank them out to our minds, but still they remain. Still there is goodness, kindness, love, beauty, fun, gentleness and pleasure, out beyond the domain of pain.

As we continue to breathe we allow these other feelings to become part of our bodies again too. We allow them to intermingle, like paint in water: the pain, the sadness, the anger, the fear, the tiredness, the despair that we have been bottling up in our muscles and minds, that have emerged and intensified through the lens of our illness.

What if rather than resist each sensation, we seep into it, allowing each to merge into the next?

What if we surrender to this flow of undifferentiated feeling, trusting that it will not erase us, but will simply wash away the dry old shells that tried to contain it?

When we do so, we realise that our suffering is just a drop in the ocean of the world's suffering. We are not the only ones suffering. Our suffering is not everything.

Our pain is just one tiny portion of the world's pain. And our pain is only a drop of our total experience in this lifetime.

If rather than long for an end time, we let go of the clock and slip into this very moment. And inhabit it now, as fully as we can. Just this one moment has to be gotten through. Or floated through. Or breathed through. And felt. At last.

Not through self-punishment or sacrifice, guilt or martyrdom, but just because this is, for now, our life, our multifaceted drop of the world's experience to feel. Our gift to this moment is to feel it. That is all it has been waiting for, all this time: to be fully felt. To be fully known. After a lifetime of waiting.

What would happen then?
The time for resistance has passed.
Surrender to this moment at last.
At its heart lies a gem of knowledge
Can you take it on your tongue?
Can you swallow its wisdom
And allow its medicine to flow through you?

BEING SEEN

He sat across from me at my kitchen table, having driven through the snow to get to me. Having listened for several hours. This respected clinical psychologist told me what he saw, what he heard. He named my bodymind. At last. At last.

I wasn't imagining things. My brain really was different. My experiences were real. I had Asperger Syndrome. As I had suspected. The anxiety and depression stemmed from that, from trying to function in a world that wasn't built for folks like me. A world that was inherently stressful for a neurodivergent brain. He told me that it wouldn't have been discovered when I was a girl, because back then they didn't think girls tended to be high functioning autistic. It was a male thing. The diagnostic picture had been based on boys. They had only bothered diagnosing the disruptive boys, not the good girls who weren't causing a problem. Despite that fact that I was, so many of us were, struggling to navigate a world we didn't understand. Wearing a mask in public. Suffering in private.

And then he asked me how I felt. What it meant to me.

I wept as I told him of my relief, having finally, after a lifetime of knowing that something was wrong, to know what it is. To know who I was. To be heard, to be seen. To be believed.

To know that in fact, there was nothing 'wrong' at all. Nothing to be fixed. Nothing to be feared. Just plenty to be understood, a different filter to know myself through.

My soul thanked his for this sacred naming, written out in terms the System would finally understand and believe. There was little on offer in terms of healing from the System. Of course. The label didn't bring a cure. But it brought certainty, self-knowledge and hopefully understanding. It meant I could create my own way forward, access the resources I needed based on a solid foundation, not speculation, trial and error.

And with it the other physical labels, some that had been formally diagnosed, others that were self-diagnosed, fit like the pieces of the puzzle sliding into place. These illnesses that cluster together, like folks sharing an umbrella in a downpour: joint hypermobility, probably EDS type three, irritable bowel and chronic fatigue syndrome. There were no magic bullets. No cures for it all. But there were approaches I could now try.

I was home at last. Within myself. The mask of *fine* could drop forever. I could finally stop trying to outrun my fear. A new reality had been born that I could inhabit as my life. I could take the pressure off myself to be normal, to keep up with the world. I could come out as myself. I could name my reality in a language others could understand. I could find my place in my community based on my physical and mental abilities. I could seek out and weave together my own path to wellness. I could live a different way. One that worked for my body, my brain.

And I could model what this looked like for my daughter.

Finally I had the permission I had needed all my life.

In the place where doubt had lived, now there was belief: internal and external.

With this naming I had a map, a community, resources at my fingertips. I could embody the truth: my truth. I could at last live as myself.

The healing could, at long last, begin.

MEDICINE QUESTIONS

Soul

What does 'soul' mean to you?

How has this book impacted your understanding of what soul means? How has it contradicted what you believe?

Care

Do you feel cared for? When you are 'well'? When you are 'sick'?

What does feeling cared for look like to you?

Do you receive this? Are you entitled to it?

How do you ensure you are cared for? What do you have to do to access care: beg, plead, exaggerate, cry, demand? Or do you cover up and deny your needs? Or is it given without asking, are your needs anticipated?

How unwell do you have to be to qualify for care? What do you do until then? Is there a limit on the care you receive – internal or external? Does it come with conditions? What are these? Are they explicit or implicit?

Does receiving care make you feel weak, infantilised or dependent? Does it cause others to treat you as disabled or less than?

Who do you embody or channel when you care for yourself?

Is there frustration, resentment, limitation, indulgence, deep love, sensitivity or compassion in your caring for yourself? In your care for others? Do you find it easier to care for others than receive care yourself? Does caring for others help you to feel powerful or more capable or competent?

How easy do you find it to rest?

What brings you comfort?

What support do you ache for?

What nourishes you? Do you allow yourself to have this regularly?

How good an advocate are you for your own health? How has this changed since you got sick?

Perceptions of illness

How do you conceive of your illness? Do you see it as alien/an invader/foreign to you/to be defeated/as Other to the Real You? Do you see it as neutral, neither good nor bad? Do you see it as a teacher/integral to you/a gift (from life/God...)? Do you consider your suffering to be a punishment, test, spiritual trial or karma? If so, what is its message? What is its lesson? How are you learning it?

Do you consider it bad luck? Is it your fault?

Do you consider illness as meaningful in general? Has it been meaningful to you or any family members?

Or perhaps you consider it several or even all of these, depending on mood, your place on your journey. How and why does this change for you?

How do you react if others perceive it/speak of it in a different way (i.e. you see it as an unwelcome invader, and someone says it's a gift from God...)?

Does how you perceive it mirror your feelings about your body?

Does how you perceive it change your experience of it... or your symptoms?

Healing

Where do you think healing comes from?

Have you previously believed healing to be the same as curing? How do they differ?

What is needed for healing to happen?

What impact do our beliefs have on our healing?

Which aspects of healing does Western medicine provide, and which does it not provide?

Where or how can you access these missing pieces?

HEALING ARTS

Letting Go – A Ceremony

What can you let go of – in terms of unhealthy beliefs, habits, addictions, excess commitments, stressors? What support do you need to allow you to do this? What can you not let go of? What would it take to make you drop that too? Do you want that to happen?

How can you remember the parts of your bodymind that are passing away? How would it feel to create a ceremony, a grieving ritual or funeral for the self you are letting go of, where you give thanks for all that she was and did?

You may want to bury or burn something of hers. You may get rid of belongings from your past life and clear your physical space, passing on the things you no longer want or need to those who can and will treasure them. You may want to write this self a letter, poem or eulogy. You may want to pick flowers for her, gather a selection of her greatest achievements, photos of her happiest memories. Express your gratitude for her life. Express your grief at her loss. Express your hidden feelings for her, your relief at her passing, an end to her suffering. Is there anyone you want to invite to share this experience with you?

As You Are

Art projects on the subject of your body can be powerful transformative tools. In this exercise, you reclaim your body as it actually is: its power, beauty, strength, vulnerability, uniqueness through your creativity. Possibilities include:

◌ Self-portraits of your face or body in a variety of styles and media.

◌ Take a photograph each day which truly reflects your inner world.

◌ Write a love letter to your body.

◌ Dance.

◌ Sculpt your body in clay.

◌ Chart your cycles to get an inner snapshot of your body each day.

A New Relationship with Your Body

*My body was a burden. I saw it as something that unfortunately had
to be maintained. I had little patience for its needs.*
Eve Ensler, *In the Body of the World*

How do you relate to this quote? Is it true for you? Is your body a
burden? What metaphor would you use to show how it feels to inhabit
your sick body? Is it like pushing a rock up a hill, carrying a heavy
weight in your arms, a large back pack, wearing an ill-fitting suit, being taken over by an alien force, being invaded or tortured? What is
your physical experience of inhabiting your body? Can you express it
through words and images?

Once you have done this, reflect on how you would like your new relationship with your body to be – a friendship, partnership, complete
unity, a loving mother? How would you like to conceive of your body
now? Perhaps a designer outfit, a magical entity, your most treasured
possession, a temple, a cherished friend, a nature reserve... Can you
express it through words and images? What can you create or buy to
remind you of this new relationship? Perhaps a ring, a photograph,
a quotation, an amulet that you wear, carry with you or put on your
altar space. How can you build and develop this understanding in the
years to come?

I invite you to devote regular time to creating an interactive dialogue
practice with your bodymind through your creativity – this might look
like image making, writing, internal dialogue, journeying, journaling – get
into the habit of asking your bodymind what is real for it right now, what
messages it has for you and what it needs you to hear.

Finding a Great Healing Ally (for You)

What makes you trust a healing ally? (What qualities or qualifications
do you look for?)

What makes you distrust a healing ally? (What are your red flags or
immediate Nos?)

What power do you hold within your current healing relationships? Are you able to communicate when things are not working for you or when misunderstandings have occurred?

What is your attitude to medication? Which medications do you trust, and which are no-go? How do you decide?

To what extent do you trust your instincts/intuition or body knowing? How has this evolved or changed over the course of your life? What changed?

What caused you to change 'allegiance'? What is it you look for to trust?

What are things you distrust? Why?

Often we can find it hard to pick new therapists or doctors, it can seem pretty overwhelming. Sometimes we use the phone book or Google, other times we ask for recommendations. These are all great ways of finding information, but how do we know that what they offer will be a good fit for our personality, individual needs and budget?

Answer the questions above and make use of the ratings system over the page. From the responses you give create a checklist for yourself. Then the next time you are looking for a healing ally or considering changing allies, you have an easy reference list for yourself.

FINDING A HEALING ALLY. WHAT'S IMPORTANT TO ME?

Rate 1-10 (10 being the most important):

PERSONAL RECOMMENDATION	1 · 2 · 3 · 4 · 5 · 6 · 7 · 8 · 9 · 10
PRICE	1 · 2 · 3 · 4 · 5 · 6 · 7 · 8 · 9 · 10
PROFESSIONAL QUALIFICATIONS	1 · 2 · 3 · 4 · 5 · 6 · 7 · 8 · 9 · 10
YEARS' EXPERIENCE	1 · 2 · 3 · 4 · 5 · 6 · 7 · 8 · 9 · 10
DIVERSE EXPERIENCE	1 · 2 · 3 · 4 · 5 · 6 · 7 · 8 · 9 · 10
GENDER	1 · 2 · 3 · 4 · 5 · 6 · 7 · 8 · 9 · 10
PROXIMITY TO HOME/ WORK/EASE OF TRAVEL	1 · 2 · 3 · 4 · 5 · 6 · 7 · 8 · 9 · 10
ETHOS	1 · 2 · 3 · 4 · 5 · 6 · 7 · 8 · 9 · 10
TECHNIQUES USED	1 · 2 · 3 · 4 · 5 · 6 · 7 · 8 · 9 · 10
WAITING LIST	1 · 2 · 3 · 4 · 5 · 6 · 7 · 8 · 9 · 10
NICHE EXPERIENCE	1 · 2 · 3 · 4 · 5 · 6 · 7 · 8 · 9 · 10
INSTITUTION STUDIED AT	1 · 2 · 3 · 4 · 5 · 6 · 7 · 8 · 9 · 10
ABILITY TO LISTEN	1 · 2 · 3 · 4 · 5 · 6 · 7 · 8 · 9 · 10
COMPASSIONATE	1 · 2 · 3 · 4 · 5 · 6 · 7 · 8 · 9 · 10
FEELS SAFE	1 · 2 · 3 · 4 · 5 · 6 · 7 · 8 · 9 · 10

HEALING THE FEMININE

We have taken a whole entire part of life and have oppressed it. The masculine principle is saying that the feminine principle of beauty, shining one's light and being a presence in the world and tapping into deep knowing and deep listening is not okay. And it's creating huge illness. It's affecting our emotional health, our physical health, because it's all connected. It's affecting the health of the planet.
Sandra Ingerman, in *Femme: Women Healing the World*

To help heal a body or mind and leave the soul unattended is only doing part of the healer's work. Women's healing is often coupled with ritual. Ritual speaks to the 'deep mind' – the spirit within – in the language of symbols ...[and] communicates the possibility of change to our spirit-selves...
Jade River, *To Know*

The knowledge of our fathers has been gifted to us through the culture of patriarchy, but the wisdom of our mothers has been lost. Our appreciation for the masculine body and Father god has been cultivated to the entire exclusion of the divine Feminine and the powers of a woman's body. Tales of soul have been replaced with the knowledge of the mind. Masculine ways of knowing have entirely supplanted women's ways, labelling them old wive's tales.

Women's spiritual, biological and psychological needs – in short the foundations of women's health – have been lost, ignored and sidelined over hundreds of years. In a System that emphasises product over process, the major (and distinctly female) body transformations of menarche, menstruation, birth and menopause, as well as the human processes of illness, death and psychological and spiritual development have not been considered meaningful. The power and intelligence of the body and the need of the soul to be celebrated and supported in their growth have been overlooked, numbed and controlled. Any sense of agency, power or achievement have been stripped from them. The Feminine – the tides of hormones, the dance of muscular contractions and releases, the movements of the soul as expressed through the female body has been repressed and denied.

No wonder we are sick now.

Medicine Woman calls us to bring forward the long-suppressed Feminine aspects of healing. She shows us that at the heart of women's healthcare must be rooted a multi-level understanding of, and respect for, our female bodymind's function: an understanding which is shared, supported and nurtured by the culture we inhabit.

The distinct self-care, knowledge, community involvement and mentoring needed to be a healthy woman, which should be our birthright, are thankfully being reclaimed as a matter of urgency by different individuals and communities around the world. We are piecing them together. For ourselves. For our daughters. For our mothers. And for our sisters who are not yet sick from the System, who are still unaware how much of what they are needing has been denied, withheld or deemed unnecessary.

A woman's ability to intercede with spirit and to heal the body have always been tied up together. To paraphrase Merlin Stone, the disappearance of women's rights happened at the same time as the disappearance of her rites. This has been the basic goal of patriarchy since time immemorial: remove a woman's authority within herself, within her community, remove her right to speak for herself or others, remove her ways of healing and knowing, shame her direct relationship with her body, the cycles of nature and the Greater Mystery, remove the Feminine from all and in its place supplant your own unquestionable authority, your own beliefs and systems. On pain of death. Or just on pain.

But it is because of this pain that we are now learning the urgency of rebalancing and reconnecting our female systems to the Feminine after our enforced life-long exile in the world of the toxic masculine. The agony of the masculine darkness is teaching us that we need regular descent into the inner darkness of the Feminine to stay healthy and whole. We require regular contact with our Feminine cores to stay powerful.

The life we now see as normal has been built by the minds of men, but it is being healed through the bodies of women. Unhealthy patterns have been built up over lifetimes, based on generations of beliefs and behaviours which cumulatively created the culture we now inhabit. Unlearning these old behaviours and replacing them with more health-creating practices based on new values takes time, patience, effort, energy and most of all commitment and courage to a new vision, often in the face of disbelief, ridicule and a lack of understanding.

We are learning intimately what it means to inhabit a woman's body, not how it *should* be. We are learning how to exist on this planet, at *this* time, *in* our bodies, rather than within a numbed, performed persona. We are learning how to stay here as ourselves, in our full, real, broken, messy bodyminds. We are learning – and teaching – not to powerlessly accept suffering as our duty, but find ways to heal and transform it. Learning how to make it better. For us all.

At the crux of the treatment of women's illness in patriarchy is the inherent belief of woman's body being weak and her mind being unreliable. In time we believe these things of ourselves.

As we learn to listen to our bodies, as we feel our feelings, an old voice will probably emerge.

Isn't this awfully self-indulgent?

Oh boohoo, you've been crying forever and not gotten anywhere.

Pull yourself together. Snap out of it. Get on with it.

Stop being a wuss.

What will people think?

Just get better already.

Everyone will think you are crazy.

This is the shadow masculine, the inner critic, the internalised patriarch. The one who we swallowed down with our mother's milk as we learned not to make a fuss, not to cry. We have been taught that being brave meant keeping everything inside, and not upsetting other people.

From a young age we have been told stories of the Crazy Woman and what happens to her. We have been taught since childhood to tune out the communications of our own bodies. To override the inner voice. To silence our own illness and pain.

We have become deeply deficient in the Feminine.

Deeply deficient in ourselves.

....

My physical depletion comes partly from my diet which itself is lacking because we've over-farmed the Earth and depleted her soil. My emotional depletion likewise came from a society where mothers are not well supported and hurting children was acceptable.
So yes, [my illness is] a great teacher even on bad days as it's making me re-evaluate my work-life balance and put me first, probably for the first time ever. It coincides so perfectly with perimenopause, when we are meant to pause and take stock. I really wouldn't have stopped without my illness. I see it as opening up new opportunities for me in the future, which I would never have discovered if I spent the rest of my working life serving others.
I detest feeling so weak and dependent but there are deep lessons for me here too. It feels like getting the care I should have received as a child – so healing.

JOY

....

All that we have suppressed, intentionally and unintentionally, is coming to the surface for breath, for transformation, coming to consciousness for healing. All that has festered in the shadows is emerging. This is happening both in our own personal lives and bodies, and on a community scale. It is so vast that we cannot ignore it any longer. It is so big and scary that we regularly still wish we could.

As it tries to emerge we can find our Feminine energy blocked by the old, toxic masculine, trapped in old ways of being, old habits, old behaviours, trapped by the sick culture. To heal we need to find ways to free it. Through dance and art and orgasm and telling our stories we liberate our Feminine energy from the binds of the internalised patriarchy, from our fear of *what if* – to ground it once more, to centre it within our bodies, to live by it, to allow it to run through us and power our daily lives.

WOMAN HEALING

*Women healers long ago were known as witches, a word that came from Old English **witan**, which meant 'to know' or 'to be wise'.*
Barbara Tedlock

When we refuse the shame and victimhood that comes with sickness and reclaim our right and ability to heal, when we choose to step out in radical authenticity, embodying the fullness of ourselves, the intricate weaving of our pain and love, darkness and light, we step into the archetype of Woman Healing.

Woman Healing is she who has committed healing on her own terms, she who is learning to walk between the worlds. She is an edgewalker, a wayshower, a pioneer, a changemaker, a transformer, a shapeshifter, a woman always becoming. She is a heroine, a priestess, a wise woman, a witch.

She is me.

She is you.

Woman Healing begins to see that life is wilder, more chaotic, harsher and more loving, paradoxical, and downright strange than she was ever taught. She discovers for herself the pull of the moon, the shifting of the seasons, the haze of pollen and fall in air pressure and how they intimately impact her dreams, her moods, her body processes, her blood and bones. She learns that she is not an independent automaton but a wild being woven of life and death: a chaos of magic, not a machine of logic. She learns that the outer impacts the inner in myriad ways. And vice versa. She learns that she is simultaneously weaker and yet more powerful than she ever knew. She is dangerous because of this inner knowing, which does not appear in the medical books and bibles except as anomalies. She is singing from the wrong hymn sheet and messing up the patina of perfection that the patriarchy is aiming for with her body. In a display of a million marching soldiers with polished boots, gleaming medals and straight legs, there is the sick woman, bare-breasted, hair loose, scars showing, shameless, dancing to her own tune, resting on their time. In a land run on adrenaline, she is learning to transform her energy source.

Woman Healing knows that her existence is at odds with the productive society she inhabits. Her views are marginalised because she is marginal. But she is dangerous because she is contagious – she has too much time on her hands, she thinks too much, she sees behind the façade of the healing/spiritual complex. She asks awkward questions and proves their certainty wrong with the reality of her bodymind. She casts a shadow over the certainty and knowledge that they profess to. She refuses to pay their price with her life. She is writing a new story with her own blood.

Woman Healing has moved from feeling alienated, detached from her body, alone in the world, to finding a home and identity within it again, expanding her sense of self far beyond what she has previously understood it to be. She is learning day by day to trust herself as a respected authority and finds others whose authority she trusts. She is healing through developing a new caring, living, working partnership between her body and soul. Using the medicines of the world, and the medicines of the soul, she pours her energy into creating an interconnected, ensouled body and an embodied soul, understanding both as sacred.

....

I see my symptoms as a sign that I am a pioneer, and that I am so aligned with my soul/natural balance/truth that my system reacts to the fact that society, ideals, media, patriarchal ideas are rotten and harmful for all of us.
I see all of us women who suffer as prophet voices that call out that something is very, very wrong in the way we as society live... the way we live with the Earth, the way we live with each other, the way we live with our bodies and souls.
I really see us as brave truth tellers... like the elders of the tribe, telling the truth with our bodies. And I don't need the confirmation or approval from others of my view. I know we humans are all out of whack... and I feel that women who abandon what has been told to them about health/balance/sexuality/love/body image/femininity and spirituality and who go on a quest to find a truer truth... are the pioneers of this era. And I think the future will give us more women who can actually chart symptoms and illnesses and the imbalances that they point to, in order to bring back a higher balance, that doesn't just

focus on making us able to take on a full-time job. But this takes a shift in our way of seeing ourselves when we are sick, so that we don't see ourselves as damaged goods, but as pioneers and brave souls that can restore the waste land of the modern civilization.

ANNA

Woman Healing understands through her lived experience that her body has power and life of its own – and that it is her sacred duty to stay connected to this and honour it. She recognises that she cannot mentally leave her body as a form of escape from her illness or the perceived dangers of the world for very long and remain healthy. Instead of trying to control life with her mind, the Woman Healing learns to feel into her body, come fully into her body and live from this place. This is where she can access and root her power.

Woman Healing treasures the visions she receives in her fevers, her dreams, her hallucinations and learns not to dismiss their weird wisdom. She journeys to places that our culture fears most. Illness gives her the circumstances to journey deep into the inner world and far beyond and to come back with her own medicine.

Woman Healing learns firsthand how fear can transform any experience for the worst. She learns in the darkness of night and the depths of her pain to reach for and lean into the arms of a higher power, a greater spirit than her own. She learns the power of love to transform.

Woman Healing understands that nurturing her own health is not an optional extra but crucial to her wellbeing. She knows that care and self-care are central to her role as woman – that a vital aspect of the Feminine is caretaker: caring for ourselves, our bodies, our families, our communities, our Earth. She understands that care is valuable, important work that must be prioritised, supported by the Masculine, not undermined or overridden by it. She learns too that not only female bodies are responsible for caring or feeling: it must be shared. The Feminine and Masculine must at last come together in and through *all* our bodies. We must all learn how to care.

Woman Healing re-members that she is not a victim of her circumstances but has agency. She advocates for herself, asking for what she needs, speaking her experience clearly without drama. She understands the spirals of drama and negativity and how they can create their own forces. She understands the power of positivity too, not a false positivity but one that looks for and focuses on what there is to be grateful for, even on the darkest of days. She recognises the power and danger of the inner critic. She gives thanks each and every day. And remembers her power to transform or accept that which is objectionable to her.

Woman Healing is an active participant in her own healing, and whilst self-care is front and centre of her life, she learns that she is not alone and cannot do it alone. She may find many allies and modalities along the path. Some for a day, others for a season. She can access the knowledge and cures of Western medicine through books and the internet, through doctors and hospitals, operations and medications. But she also knows that she is not limited by her conscious mind. She has many ways of knowing. She can move into her body for wisdom, into nature for its healing properties. She can tap into the wisdom beyond her individual soul, root into the wisdom of the Earth, she can access the wisdom of the collective unconscious, the source wisdom.

Woman Healing is no longer a passive patient, she gives her consent even in the process of surrendering to the healing actions of others.

Woman Healing understands and engages the power of community to heal, nurture, support and comfort. She builds and engages with healing community as a core part of her own health.

But she always remembers that whilst medicine women can be found without,

Medicine Woman

Lies within.

CARING FOR OURSELVES

The path to personal power requires that we know what we are called to heal and what we are not called to fix… only the willing undertaking of responsibility, can lead to healing… as women and men of conscience at the beginning of the twenty-first century, we are called to develop those qualities of courage and responsibility that can lead to healing.
Starhawk and Hilary Valentine, *The Twelve Wild Swans*

Healing starts and ends with a solemn commitment to care for ourselves as we would for a loved one, to acknowledge and honour the body's needs instead of overriding them with the mind, or the rules of others. For many of us that means breaking a lifelong unconscious agreement to punish and dissociate ourselves from our physical bodies. We learn to move from body as enemy to befriending, trusting and listening to our bodies even when – especially when – they are weak, ailing or broken. Before the body can become a temple for the Feminine, first it must become our very human home.

Women's work has always been to care, but historically it has been for other people... and for our homes. Self-care in terms of maintaining our appearance – grooming, shaving, dying our hair, toning our bodies – is a cultural condition of acceptance for women, required for the performance of the feminine, our social acceptance and sexual attractiveness. Without these the female body in its natural state is deemed unacceptable, disgusting even. But maintaining our inner health, our connection to our innate Feminine wellbeing – meh – pure indulgence and hippie claptrap.

Emotional and physical self-care have been denied the adult female population historically and systematically. Unless it has been commodified. Within capitalist society our basic needs have been codified as luxury goods to be earned or deserved. 'Me time' and 'pampering' are things we get as a reward after a long day or once a year as a gift, packaged and sold back to us as products: the expensive candle or bath oil, the birthday spa day, the fancy massage, the manicure. We do not have the time or the cultural permission to integrate deep self-care – rather than superficial appearance maintenance – into our lives.

....

I see my painful joints and digestive illnesses as the symptoms of the culmination of stress and trauma in my system. Through my recent training I have realised that my autonomic nervous system is to use the Irish expression 'banjaxed' – a lifetime of inner fear/terror/not feeling safe combined with repressed emotions and strong patterns of 'trying so hard' and 'holding it together'. I am so exhausted from holding it together! So, in a way I see my symptoms as a journey to acknowledging my story, an exploration of my history, the effects of

my lineage and an opportunity to slow down, to pause, to soften my
armour, to include myself – not to focus on meeting other's needs
(read, my kids') always over my own – to practise self-compassion.
I believe for me (and for many others) the initial wound was in the
relational and the healing is also in the relational, so I take baby steps
in being truly seen, in showing my vulnerability and in trusting that
I will not be rejected.

MICHELLE

For a woman to claim time to herself, for interiority, to take time to dedicate to her body, to live according to her inner rhythms and needs, to dedicate time to healing herself is revolutionary: it breaks with centuries-old dictums that a woman's time is not her own, her energy is not her own, her body is not her own. It contradicts the unwritten energetic contract that your female energy should be solely dedicated to the care of others, that you are not worthy of care.

Caring for ourselves requires the outrageous belief that we are worth caring for.

You, my dearest love, are so deeply worthy of care.

Do you know this?

I became gentler, and more compassionate – with myself and others. I
gave myself a long-awaited and needed break, time out from a hectic,
passionate, energetic (non-stop) career. I went through some difficult
mental, emotional and physical processes, but found new depths and
parts of myself that I never could have without being ill. While I had a
fever for three days, I had dreams and stories that began to form when
I was in-between sleep and consciousness. Characters for a new book
began to emerge and taught me to be connected to animals, the natural
world and my imagination. Coupled with my shamanic training and
meditation, it opened up a whole new way of seeing and being in the
world, and my place in it.
I know that one thing I did not appreciate was people telling me – and
there were some – to 'cheer up'. I did not feel 'down', I was simply

going through what I had to, and I could not run from it. I had run around – literally, as I am an active person by nature, and figuratively from something that had happened to me in my teenage years – all my life, but this time, no – I would have to learn to rest, and to look after myself. My illnesses were going to teach me how. Had it not been for them I would have continued on, often struggling, weak, exhausted. I found it, in this way, a strange blessing but difficult to articulate. This spilled over into my writing, and I gained a new book that I felt helped me in my own personal growth. The women in my dreams spilled over into my waking life where I would suddenly have flashes of the next part of their story. They were as real to me as though they sat beside me, and in this way they began to tell me their stories. I would never have gone to such depths had I not been as ill as I was.

CIARA

Major illness often reawakens memories of what it felt like to be cared for – or not – as a child. We often lose our abilities to care for ourselves, finding that we must rely on others to feed, wash, dress and drive us. We can often find ourselves reverting to childish habits and feelings. It is a time, in the midst of our physical healing, to begin to heal these long held hurts. Often we can only begin to do this through the modelling of new health-creating behaviours from healing allies, as we develop a different understanding of what it feels like to receive and accept care. We begin, perhaps for the first time, or in a new way, to learn to care for ourselves, to step into the role of our own carers in a healthier way.

As we begin to regain our autonomy we learn that the acts of self-care are not luxuries, as we have been taught by our culture, they are vital practices: living, breathing rituals to sustain and nurture bodymind and soul. Self-care is rarely glamorous and often depends on how much energy we have. On a good day it looks like eating food that fully nourishes our bodyminds, but some days it is just being able to eat something and keep it down. Some days it is walking a mile, other days it is being able to get out of bed for a minute and raise our arms in the air to stretch. A vital part of self-care is learning how to adapt our practices to our differing daily needs, rather than letting self-care be another stick we use to beat ourselves with. Self-care is there to care for us. Not add to our guilt or feeling of disability. It looks and feels different each day. But at its core it is a commitment to finding healthy ways to nurture ourselves independently. To focus on our health and wellbeing as a sacred practice, rather than an optional extra. It is to learn, at last, at last, to centre ourselves in our own lives, to learn to live to our own rhythm. Through our self-care we rediscover how to recharge, replenish and retreat as regular practices, we learn how to consciously support our bodyminds in their process of regulation, rather than endlessly fighting or ignoring them.

I have discovered that using the different elements of fire, water, earth and air to focus my self-care practices helps me to choose more easily what I need. I am not a person who has a consistent practice which looks the same every day. Using these elemental prompts helps me to focus on what feels out of balance in my body and therefore how I might balance this within myself.

- Fire (in need of stillness, warmth, comfort or inner passion): having some time by candlelight, an open fire, a warming drink, a bonfire, cooking a pot of nourishing soup, time in the sun.

- Water (cleansing, purifying, releasing, lack of fluidity or flow, racing mind, needing to be calmed and held): a swim or paddle in the sea, lake, river or pool, a bath or shower, a big drink of water or herbal tea, watching a waterfall or fountain, facial steam or sauna.

- Air (feeling trapped, stuck, longing for freedom): going for a walk, run or dance, feeling the wind in your hair, the air on your skin, opening windows, breathing practices.

- Earth (feeling ungrounded, detached, lack of solidity, panicky): moulding clay, planting and harvesting in a garden or flower pot, walking barefoot on sand or mud, having a picnic on the grass, collecting pebbles or shells, balancing rocks.

- Colour (feeling grey, disillusioned, drained): soaking in the colours you feel drawn to, a walk in a wood or garden for green, by the sea for blue, to a gallery for multi-colours, painting with or wearing a certain colour.

- Silence (exhausted, overwhelmed, buzzing): taking time for the bodymind to settle and absorb the medicine of stillness and silence through meditation, sitting still, reading contemplatively, watching nature.

◯ Expression (trapped energy, going in circles): seeing a therapist, talking to a friend, making art, writing in your journal, having nourishing sexual experience, singing, dancing or screaming.

◯ Depletion: rest, sleep, meditation, nutritious food and supplements.

Self-care practices are what help us to reach and maintain the equilibrium of our psyche and our soma, our bodymind. They help our biological and spiritual selves to move from aligning with the endemic dysregulation of the man-made world, into a regulated inner state which is in harmony with, not at odds with, our inner natures and Nature herself.

CYCLE WISDOM

Turbulence teaches grounding.
The edge teaches breath.
Falling teaches rising.
Breaking teaches building.
Pain teaches healing.
Resentment teaches boundaries.
Failing teaches rebirth.
Harmony continuously seeks itself.
Remember, it is simply a circle continuing on,
and you are supported.
Victoria Erickson, *Rhythms & Roads*

Western culture runs by clock time and calendrical dates, man-made ways of slicing up our lived experience, so that we live by an externally imposed schedule, rather than our internal rhythms. Although clocks and calendars are ostensibly based around the revolutions of the Earth, they are actually dictated by the System: we finish work when our boss says we are done, not when it is dark, or when we are tired or hungry.

We have become so used to treating our bodies as though they were machines and considering ourselves independent of nature. But we are not.

We are in fact intimately embedded within natural cycles of growth and renewal, decay and death. But we have learned to ignore or deny this. Our bodyminds are subject to solar and lunar gravitational pulls, radiation and light levels and so many other natural phenomena that our conscious minds are unaware of, but which impact our biological selves on a continual basis. Each of these natural phenomena tend to work on a cyclical basis, the length of the cycle ranging from mere microseconds, to daily, annual or even longer.

For most of our evolutionary history humans would have unconsciously responded to these cycles and lived their lives in harmony with them. However, the definition of late-stage modernity is the over-riding of pretty much all of our natural rhythms with the mind: staying awake long into the night, taking the contraceptive pill, eating the same foods all year round, being on the go all the time, travelling fast over time zones.

On top of this the environmental cycles themselves are shifting from their natural balance because of man's impact, with seasons and weather shifting to bi-polar extremes. To get back to health our bodies need to find their own inner equilibrium once more, as well as to harmonise with, rather than fight against the bio-cycles that they have intelligently evolved in response to. To enable them to do this in this unbalanced world environment, we need to consciously and constantly reconnect to them.

Why? Because our bodies have natural healing states built into them cyclically. The most obvious for all of us being the nightly sleep cycle. But most women's bodies have further cycles built in. Menstruation and the post-partum period are two of the most obvious. At these times they enter a different state of consciousness, releasing the toxins and toxic emotions from the previous cycle, resting deeply, and allowing for the regeneration of tissues and the psyche. Or rather they do if we allow them.

As a culture we ignore these recovery periods, and label them as times of weakness and taboo. Our attitude towards them combines our distaste for the Feminine, for sickness, bodies and death. Whereas actually they are a core part of the body's innate healing mechanism. As are the times when we are bedridden with illness, delirious with fever, exhausted or depressed. Our bodies detach us from calendar and clock time, sequestering us from busyness, enforcing a break with daily life, allowing the mind and body to be still and enter the more trance-like state of consciousness necessary for healing.

If we can allow ourselves to understand illness therefore not as something wrong or a dangerous aberration of nature but rather as a necessary part of the cycle, then we can understand how and why it may occur in our lives, rather than fighting it. Indeed, many of the chronic conditions that women struggle with have cyclical relapses: MS, fibromyalgia, migraine, depression and joint issues tend to flare with stress, hormonal shifts and seasonal changes.

Learning to live by both our inner female rhythms and the outer bio-rhythms is vital for our health as women. We are staying sick because we are disconnected from our innate life-cycles and engaged instead with the life-denying, destructive-cycles of patriarchal culture. When we reconnect with the Feminine, with the cycles of nature within and outside of us, our bodies shift into life-affirming cycles once more. Once the flow state is re-established, once the physical and emotional blocks to it have been removed, our healing response can unfold naturally.

When our bodyminds become stressed they are disrupted. Whilst many of us have the power to choose what to take into our bodies in terms of food, water, medication and exercise to help them to find balance, we cannot eliminate all the things that stress our bodies and shift them into flare up cycles. Change is the one constant of life. Our hormones will shift as we move through our menstrual cycles and as we navigate menopause and post-partum recovery. The stresses of work, family, our culture will impact us. The shift in season will impact us. We can mitigate these effects by taking HRT or an antidepressant, not reading the news, moving to a warm country for the winter or leaving our families. But to heal more fully our narrative about change has to transform internally. We have to learn to experience ourselves as participants in relation to its creative potential, rather than experiencing ourselves as powerless victims of it.

When we move from the sense of our failure within the Hero's journey narrative, we can reclaim the image of the spiral or cycle as the Feminine shape of our journey. These symbols acknowledge that we travel through health (life) phases and dark (death) phases, just as the Earth does through the seasons. Each has a time and a place, each will come again. Some winters will be long, dark, cold and hard, and will take all our resources and energy just to survive them. Some of them will be mild. But winter will come again. We will enter the darkness once more. Its coming does not mean failure. It does not mean certain death. It is time for another letting go, another period of resting and release, the acceptance of a time of no apparent outer growth, a time when life goes underground.

Our female bodyminds are meant to move gracefully between our many different realms of being and our natural cycles are there to ensure this. Our brains are designed to cycle between different states of consciousness: alpha, beta, theta and delta states. They are made to shift regularly between trance, REM sleep, light sleep, meditation, flow consciousness, as well as hyper focus, relaxed awareness and play. They are built to discharge upset and imbalance physically and emotionally at the time of its occurrence. But instead within our culture this natural urge is suppressed.

Our bodyminds are not supposed to be jammed into the high adrenaline, fight or flight mode that suppresses our nervous systems and routine biological cycles. The parasympathetic nervous system is supposed to kick in right after high alert to calm and heal us. But patriarchal society requires endless adrenaline-fuelled hyper-arousal, denying the trauma that is accumulated along the way in the process, giving no tools or opportunity for detoxification. We continue until we collapse. And then wonder what went wrong.

Our current System is based on adrenaline. The other possibility is built on maximising the release of oxytocin – the hormone of love, healing, nurturing and connection. We have both in our systems. We are equally as capable of producing either. But biologically we cannot produce both at the same time.

Adrenaline is infectious – just as oxytocin is. When others around us are pumping it out, those around them pick up on it, and respond biochemically. We have the potential for both. But our systems within the current culture are primed for just one – adrenaline. Our neural pathways are being more and more deeply engaged with adrenaline-producing behaviours. It has become our default setting: a constant feedback loop of stress leading to adrenaline, leading to fighting or hiding, leading to more adrenaline and perhaps trauma, which leads to hypervigilance, which leads to more stress and so the loop continues. And it started while we were in the womb, continued during birth, and on, and on… childhood traumas, school, exams, financial stress, conflicts, illness. Our systems are depleted, exhausted from running on survival state permanently. We need to find and create safe space where we can rest. Where we can reconnect to our health-sustaining bio-cycles. Where our bodyminds can heal at last.

Illness, depression and breakdown are often the undesired invitation for this hormonal transition.

When a transformative process is kickstarted by physical illness, giving birth, menopause or depression, we get the opportunity to step out of our man-made life and into a new way of being. We naturally begin living by our body's own cycles rather than clock time. We sleep a lot. Precipitated by this inner shift of consciousness, we can then start to re-order our external behaviours and the structure and contents of our lives.

This 'call to life' can sound crazy to those around us who are fully engaged with maintaining the patriarchal status quo, or rather are barely surviving in it and resenting anyone who shirks the load. Everything around us – especially medicine – is set up to reintegrate us, as quickly as possible with our old lives within the System, to find our place again within man-made rhythms of existence.

And whilst we can sustain this behaviour when stress levels inside and out are low, as they start to rise, our need to reconnect with other states of consciousness becomes a matter of life or death. When we consistently deny or annihilate this pull to the Otherworld of the soul, the other realms of consciousness, we experience a loss of life-force. And often an inability to stay alive.

So many of our health problems come from not just external stressors, but the inner stress of ignoring our biological and emotional cycles by forcing our bodyminds to fit prescribed modes of reality, rather than shaping our culture to fit our biological realities.

Our bodies are our greatest healing allies in this transformation, if we will listen, giving us constant feedback to help us to stay healthy and move towards health-making and away from disease-creating behaviours and choices.

Learning to trust the body alongside the mind, to integrate both ways of knowing goes against a lot of what we have been taught. Understanding the cycles of our lives is a biological imperative for women's health and a powerful way of making a break with patriarchal reality and connecting on a visceral level to the Feminine. When we regularly access other states of consciousness, through dreaming sleep, trance, meditation, creativity, we strengthen our ability to heal.

So how can we do this in practical terms? Those of you who have read *Moon Time* will know that for years I have been charting my menstrual cycle. Initially I did it to help me to heal my PMS and crippling period pains. Once these had resolved, it was about knowing where my body was within its own cycles so that I could navigate my own shifting energetic and emotional terrain with more grace and ease.

As I continued to dive deeper into my charting practices with *Full Circle Health* I realised that many of my physical symptoms were connected to my menstrual cycle – my joints would ache more and be more likely to dislocate in the week preceding my period and the first couple of days of my bleeding because of hormonal changes. I realised I would be more likely to get over-stressed and over-tired at this stage in my cycle, which would lead to more panic attacks and migraines. I could release the tension built up over the month at this time, but I couldn't take any more. But if I let myself rest deeply at this time, I would tend to have powerful insights and my creativity would emerge from a deeper level of my being.

I also realised that my cycles were not independent of the cycles of nature. My sleep, and that of my children, was deeply impacted by the moon's phases: on full moons we would be wired and have vivid dreams, once we eventually got to sleep. I also saw that my health tended to follow an annual cycle. Each year I would really struggle with mental health issues in June, December and February, transition points in the school year. Tonsillitis only ever hit me in mid-August. And so, I began to immerse myself deeper into observing all my physical and mental health symptoms and energy levels with curiosity to see which were cyclical and what impacted them. I formulated this into a complete, flexible system of integrated health charting which I share in *Full Circle Health*, as a practical method of observing and recording the cycles and information of both body and soul, in order to support our healing as women.

As my womanhood has unfolded, I have learned to live more to the rhythm of my children, my menstrual cycle, the phases of my mental and physical health, the seasons and moon phases. But still I find myself drawn back to living to the rhythms and expectations of a culture whose values I no longer hold, yet which controls the strings of power in the world around me, that plays the Pied Piper to the dance I feel I must do to stay alive, to stay safe.

I am learning, slowly but surely, to live by my own cycles.

To *listen* deeply and carefully to my body.

I am learning to *stop* when my body tells me to.

To take my *foot off the gas* and *nourish* myself.

To make *space* for myself,

Make *time* for myself.

To *watch* what I have been told to ignore

And *reach out* for support.

To *rest*.

I have been taking my medicine:
Art as medicine
Sex as medicine
Nature as medicine
Circles as medicine
Touch as medicine
Music as medicine
Movement as medicine
Prayer as medicine
Food as medicine
Colour as medicine
Tears as medicine
Silence as medicine
Love as medicine
Darkness as medicine.
Will you join me?

THE SPIRAL JOURNEY OF HEALING

The doors to the world of the wild Self are few but precious. If you have
a deep scar, that is a door, if you have an old, old story, that is a door...
If you yearn for a deeper life, a full life, a sane life, that is a door.
Clarissa Pinkola Estés, Women Who Run With the Wolves

At first I didn't want to start the journey of healing, because I was scared the world that I had so carefully manufactured would fall down around me if I moved any significant piece.

So I didn't start anywhere. Just kept looking for the right way in.

Round and around I went in my head, whilst my body got sicker and sicker. Round and around looking for the way in to healing.

What I didn't realise was this: there is no 'right way'. There is no one beginning point. But a thousand possible entryways.

I took just one. You may take another.

And just as there is no one beginning point, so too there is no one end point. But a different ending every moment, every day.

What I have learned is that healing has its own innate path and pattern, once it is set in motion in many ways it sets its own course and has its own internal timing. Sometimes it feels as though nothing is shifting, however much you do and change, and then suddenly something small and seemingly insignificant happens and a whole immovable edifice of suffering collapses into the ocean of non-being.

Once one part of the structure crashes down, a previously unseen one emerges. We may heal our eczema, but then realise our guts are sore and aching every day. We then start the cycle of gut healing, and when this is resolved realise that underneath it is a deep anger at our mothers, we embark on that healing journey, and reveal a deep-rooted abandonment anxiety, and a new allergy, meanwhile our eczema begins to flare again.

We heal in spirals.

The healing journey – once we start it – is a lifetime adventure whose only certain outcome is death. It is one that will shift and change as circumstances change. But once we have learned the dynamics of the spiral journey of healing, how to find healing allies, reach out beyond ourselves, form healing communities, trust our bodies, then we never have to start from ground zero again.

Until we do.

I have learned to trust this. Much as with the creative process. If you keep showing up. If you keep doing your side of the bargain, magic turns up to meet you. Not everyday. Not always. But there is an internal intelligence to the process which needs to be met by our own effort, willingness and belief. It cannot be forced but it needs to be opened to. It needs our commitment not our desperate petitions.

It needs *us* in order to work.

MIDLIFE/CRISIS

Whatever the issue, it seems as if we spend the first half of our lives shutting down feelings to stop the hurt, and the second half trying to open everything back up to heal the hurt.[113]
Brené Brown

At some point has your suffering been written down to the two patronising words: midlife crisis?

We are all too familiar with the term 'midlife crisis' especially in men. It is a term bandied about in contemporary culture, derided as an unwillingness to grow up, or a desperate second blast at youth by riding a motorbike or having an affair. With women midlife is of course associated with the menopause as a cessation of biological fertility, but not so much with the energetic transition.

In the words of Brené Brown, "midlife is not a crisis, it is an unravelling." She continues:

Midlife is when the universe gently places her hands upon your shoulders, pulls you close, and whispers in your ear: 'I'm not screwing around. All of this pretending and performing – these coping mechanisms that you've developed to protect yourself from feeling inadequate and getting hurt – has to go. Your armor is prevent-

ing you from growing into your gifts. [...] You can't live the rest of your life worried about what other people think. You were born worthy of love and belonging. Courage and daring are coursing through your veins [...] It's time to show up and be seen.[115]

Midlife is a powerful energetic transition point. As I explained in *Full Circle Health*, transition points between two phases of a cycle are places of potential crisis, but they are also places of immense transformational potential and power: as the old self falls away, we come closer to the authentic self within.

The two major windows for sickness/transformation in women seem to be the time of the move into the worldly persona – as the last vestiges of childhood fall away in late-adolescence through to the mid-twenties, and then the mental or physical collapse that often occurs in a woman's late thirties and forties. Both are biological and energetic transition points between two cycles – the transit from maiden to fertile creatrix. And the transit from fertile woman working, caring, birthing, nurturing, to the role of Wise Woman/Queen and Crone. These transitions are rarely acknowledged, let alone marked, supported or given time, space or guidance. But our souls don't care, they are demanding it through our bodies.

Our culture invests in us developing a strong and consistent persona, which is a more feasible proposition for men, whose physical and emotional selves are less carved by the procreative cycle of the fertile years. This identity that is built through our teens and early adulthood, is expected to be one that *should* contain us with as little change as possible until our physical death. But when the onset of sickness breaks this shell, the physical self becomes dis-abled in some way, whilst the soul tries to shed the old body and fit into a more spacious container for the next part of its life. Most parts of mainstream culture mitigate against this transformation, denying its necessity. The harder we try to hold it all together and return to normal, the harder the soul has to push in its birthing process which can become messy and painful, or aborted all together.

I discussed this with a trusted circle of women, who had been travelling the unravelling journey alongside me through this last long dark winter – literal and metaphorical. We had each turned to the same antidepressant in order to find a way to regain our functionality in bodyminds that were crumbling under the strain. We each had been very hesitant about medication. But were all finding it a blessed bridge back to ourselves. We reflected that it was, however, a cultural necessity for us. That in a different culture we may have been able to rest for as long as we needed, our sisters and mothers and aunts would have been around to help care for the children and the home, we would not be driving to jobs, or to afterschool clubs whilst trying to navigate this inner descent. We were honouring it as best we could, by resting and off-loading responsibilities, but in our culture being able to take an indefinite break to navigate this passage is a luxury. There was no space, no time for the fullness of descent required. The Western world does not stop for descent. Our overstretched nuclear families needed us. We had to find a way to return before we were ready, because there was no support within our wider culture for this process. There was no care for us the caregivers.

THE GIFT OF DARKNESS

There is no coming to consciousness without pain. People will do anything, no matter how absurd, in order to avoid facing their own Soul. One does not become enlightened by imagining figures of light, but by making the darkness conscious.
C.G. Jung

We need to find regular ways of both accessing, and moving through, dark liminal spaces, to experience them not as places of powerlessness, but instead of infinite potential, as training grounds for the soul.
from Burning Woman

Illness has at its heart periods of darkness, both literal and metaphorical. We sleep more, retreat from the world in our beds. We dissociate ourselves – consciously or unconsciously – from the pressures, expectations and cultural behaviours of the man-made world, and immerse ourselves in the dark chaos of biology and soul to reconnect with the most basic part of what makes us human.

Our visits to the darkness are a key part of almost any healing experience. But as a culture we do everything within our power to 'keep the lights on' figuratively and literally: our fear of the dark is existential.

In biological terms, bright light activates the neo-cortex (the newest part of the brain which is responsible for complex thought), it also stimulates adrenaline production. In safe, dark places the body produces oxytocin, melatonin and other hormones which allow access to the more primal parts of the brain and promote feelings of deep relaxation and ease and improve the physical healing response.

In *Burning Woman* I wrote extensively about the Feminine darkness as a place of healing, rest and rebirth, very different to the masculine darkness that we as women have been taught to fear. In patriarchal philosophy the dark represents the realm of death, the irrational, the chaotic – a direct threat to logic and control. We have been taught to avoid the darkness, to be afraid of it, to ignore the formless chaos of the dark in preference for the shiny order of the man-made world.

Medicine Woman leads you back to your Feminine darkness, to your bones, to die and be rebirthed. To engage with her we must overcome the innate fear of the dark Feminine within our culture. We must confront our fears: of death, feeling powerless, our deep grief at losing what we love, of change, of things being outside of our control. We must find ways to switch off the adrenaline-fuelled existence we have been conditioned to and switch over to the hormone of the Feminine: oxytocin.

Rather than avoid it, we need to facilitate 'going dark' on a regular basis – the deep rest, the inner journey, the letting go, the shedding, the reflection, the visits with Medicine Woman and to the Underworld are vital to our continued health. Rather than be the caged canary, dragged into the masculine darkness whose toxicity we cannot escape, instead we take an active role in descending regularly into the Feminine dark. Some of us need to do this more frequently if we are on a path of deep transformation in ourselves, if we come from backgrounds of fragmentation, physical or emotional trauma if we are professional healers or creatives. All of us are called underground more frequently in these transition times. We are growing more accustomed to the journey, and rather than fighting it, are learning how to traverse it more consciously.

It is no coincidence that the Feminine is associated with the darkness in part because it is its natural environment: the mysterious womb-space of birth, growth and death. And in part because the Feminine has been hidden there in the shadows, buried, dissociated from the light, from masculine reason and action.

Arriving in the darkness is a time of initiation. It is an essential part of the life-cycle for our continued growth and development. But in the darkness our vision goes, our fears can rise, the terror of being stuck here forever, of being cut off from ourselves and our world can subsume us and we panic.

But what if the dark feminine and the light masculine are more than just archetypal ideas or metaphors, but also physical realities? What if the two worlds that we move between are literal – the conscious and unconscious mind, the left and right sides of the brain, the rational and intuitive ways of knowing? What if they are activated by two different hormones, oxytocin (love, connection and relaxation) and adrenaline (excitement, fear and competitiveness) that cannot co-exist?

Whilst the medical profession engages our logical minds with theirs, to heal fully we have to engage the unconscious mind – the part of our brain that keeps us alive, heals our cells, the unseen part that the feelings and thoughts emerge from: the dark self at the centre. Our culture, based on logic, light and adrenaline has insinuated that dark is the opposite of light, if light is good then dark must be bad. A moral judgement is made: the unknown is dangerous, all our fears and superstitions are piled onto this place. We are taught to keep away from the dark because, being unknown, our rules cannot help guide us there, our paradigm does not extend to it. Therefore this *terra incognita* is to be avoided, so that it does not infect or kill us.

....

Adrift again, homeless in my car or tent, there is no place safe, no home. Unable to methylate mould toxins and chemicals (28% of the population is genetically unable to slough it off) most buildings and many places are too poisonous for me. I have environmental illness and the world is too toxic. There are hundreds of thousands like me adrift. Millions who are sick and unaware toxins are killing them. We all carry a chemical body burden and disease rates are epidemic due to the overuse of toxic chemicals. However those like me suffer weird

combinations of conditions, disabling and rendering them eventually
penniless. Many with no resources and suffering move constantly in
search of safety and in grief and hopelessness eventually commit suicide.
Danger, filth, isolation and loss are our bed-mates.
Where to go? How to survive? What to do? There is no safety net.
Some of us turn this into a searing burn of the initiate. Lost and
stripped of all pretences, naked to life, we find beauty, Goddess and
nature. One night alone in my tent, She showed up, glowing, alive. I
threw myself into writing about compassion and the sacred feminine in
form and action as the source for a vital future. Not only did this keep
me alive, it became essential and my source of hope for the future. I
speak about toxins, epidemic disease rates in children and what is hap-
pening to us and our babies, for we need to know. But my desire is to
create beauty and vitality for those like me, for all of us. This is the way.
It is time for us to know that we must change our lifestyles, habits,
become awake and live from gentle compassion to save nature as we
know it and us. I hope that I survive to see this happening. Our destiny
is to be in Eden here.

CHARLOTTE

I do not believe that the darkness is bad, any more than the dark side
of the moon is evil. It is dark because we cannot see it, we do not
understand it. It is not innately bad or wrong. Or rather we cannot
see or engage with it *until* its products emerge on the body or in the
conscious 'light' of the brain. It is only when we pick up on the direct
communications of the unconscious, the bodymind, that we have the
material we can work with and transform. The symbols, feelings, images, sensations, memories rise up like bubbles from the swamp of our
unconscious, where all things go to compost and transform. In this
model of understanding, the things that sicken us are the things that
we cannot process unconsciously, the things that need conscious help,
external support, medicine, to help break them down and digest them,
before they can be absorbed back into ourselves and into nature – before they can pass through our systems and be transformed. When too
many indigestible things accumulate we become soulfully constipated
and the toxins begin to leak out and poison our systems.

As a culture we tend to abandon those who find their way into the darkness, through genetics or accident. We blame them as weak rather than bear witness to the things that their bodyminds cannot process. We want to ignore the void, and so we ignore those who are travelling through it. It is easier that way. Easier to pretend that the darkness does not exist so that it cannot touch us. It is easier for us to deny that those who are there do not exist. To convince ourselves that their suffering is illusory. That this world is all there is, and that it is good. And so we avoid the void. We try to light-wash it, to illuminate it. We drug it. We do not share the tools or skills that we all need to navigate the void.

The world will try to keep you from the darkness. It will shackle you to the sink, the desk, it will try to keep your spirits up and keep your hands and mind busy. It will do everything in its power to keep you on the surface, and away from the dark places of your soul. But when the darkness falls know that your soul has come to claim you, so that you may know the fullness of its magnificence, the brilliance of your body and mind that the world tells you are faulty.

Within the void lies not certain death but infinite possibility, new ways forward: healing. In the void we find ourselves again, once we have been stripped of everything we use to cope, to mask, we strip off our worldly selves and find our souls once more.

It takes time and faith to let go, to keep letting go, until we are standing naked. And it takes great courage and strength to re-emerge differently. To come back. Great courage to bring with us our strange learnings, the truths that are so at odds with this shiny, fake world.

We are learning that we have to dig deep to find the roots of our sickness.

We are learning that healing lies in untangling the rootball in the dark.

GETTING STUCK

Pay attention to what they tell you to forget.
Muriel Rukeyser

Whilst the darkness is a vital part of the healing process and the void is a state we must all visit, there are times when the journey is too great for our physical or mental resources. When our systems are so over-whelmed by the enormity of the journey, when our bodyminds are completely exhausted, when the stress is inescapable we can get stuck in the darkness, in pain, despair and depression. When the seasons don't shift, we try to find a way to move the cycle on but we find that we cannot force it physically or with our wills. Sometimes we panic in this place and try to make the darkness permanent.

Often simply by breaking our inner vow of silence and inviting a trusted witness to share our darkness with us, or allowing a trusted community to hold and re-member us to ourselves, the spell of winter can be broken and new life can rise again within us. At other times it takes many different medicines for body and soul to help recalibrate our inner flow and counteract the paralysis.

This happened to me as I was trying to complete this book. After the hardest winter of my life, a winter flooded by a torrent of momentous challenges I found myself exhausted, stuck in the void.

Just like I had been stuck in the birth canal and had to be pulled headfirst by the nurses. Once again I was stuck, head first.

But this time there was no nurse.

With great irony and fierce love, Medicine Woman stood by in the shadows, as I got stuck in the void.

Recreating my genesis.

WHEN SPRING FAILS

This is the year when nothing is as it should be. A week of snow, the worst in thirty-five years, red weather warning after red warning – hurricane, blizzard, flooding – in a country with a mild climate. It is May and the farmers are only just ploughing their fields: a team of men against the clock doing what should have been done six weeks before. Crawling in formation over the belly of the Mother, their wheels slipping and getting stuck in the slickness.

I too am stuck in the mud, wheels grinding, desperately trying to find traction. My cells detected the scent of spring back in March and tried, like the tiny seeds I planted, to reach for the light, longing for summer, for new life, not this winter of a thousand deaths. But each time they leap too soon – the hailstones fall, the November winds blow in May. Those tender shoots are shocked and stunted, I bring them inside once more, I return to bed, my body shaking, brain in a whirl of fog and silent darkness.

Sink into the mud
And remember
It is made of rain and earth, tears and soil
The dead leaves that have been processed,
The rocks that have been pulverised,
It is alchemy itself, and it holds you so that you will not run away this time but will root down deeper.
Into the mud, the Earth.
Trust it and grow strong.
The water that has come from the rivers and the sea, comes down once more in your tears.
The seasons are shifting, life is returning.

I want to touch the world. I long to be in the world, of the world, once more. I want to be myself but I have lost her. I don't know how to in-habit this body – the habits that have made me have also broken me. But who am I without them? The brain I have tried to disguise has come to the fore. I have spent a life camouflaging myself in plain sight, trying to be normal, to do normal, but now that option is no longer open to me and I don't know who to be. I don't know how to live. I don't know if I can live any more.

I have never just been myself. I have never lived on my own terms. It feels dangerous. It feels like dying. It feels like my choice is my sanity or the world. I want both. But I cannot have both. I cannot do the world on the world's terms any more. I cannot single-handedly change the world, these 7 billion other diverse creatures. In my hubris I tried that too. Heck, I can't even change my family, though fuck knows I have ploughed my life energy into that. I cannot even change my own mind.

I turn death over and over in my mind as I sit in the car, rocked by the wind, lashed by the rain, watching the waves hazy through the fog crashing and crashing on the rocks.

She feels so close I can taste her. She is both tempting and terrifying. But I turn away from her and towards life once more with the last grain of energy I have.

I will have to do the only thing I have never done. Radical acceptance of myself. My limitations. And building a micro-culture where I can feel safe, where I can live as me. To send down deep roots into this mud, in the hopes that one day branches and leaves will follow. So that one day my body will be the strong trunk that can weather storms and support the weary body of my fellow traveller who needs to rest.

I discover that when I reach out my tender new branches, beyond my own fear, risking contact with what first hurt me, I am met with an amount of love my mind doesn't believe it deserves. I realise how many people hold a will for me to be here as myself, in this world, at this time. I learn that I matter.

And perhaps for the first time in my life I fully believe it.

But the fear would not stop raining down. Inside, outside, stress storms rolled in one after the other, I could not come up for breath. I was losing the strength to keep fighting. I had to be functional for my children who needed me, no other help was coming our way any time soon.

In my original birth I had been saved, in this midlife birth, it seems I must save myself, doing what I most feared: speaking out.

After two decades of refusing medication for my mind I had to give it a chance, this thing that most scared me.

After years of reading anti-psychiatry tomes and proof as to why these medicines didn't work, I had to give them a chance. Because I was stuck in the darkness, my brain was on permanent pause, I was frustrated by the fuzziness, the forgetfulness. I needed to have faith in what I didn't believe in, to help me out of the hole. I needed help to shift the fog.

One of my greatest fears is that medication will make me not myself.

I do not have one bit of judgment about my child who needs insulin because their body cannot make it. I do not judge myself for taking a vitamin tablet because my body does not get all its nutrients from the depleted foods I eat. I do not judge my partner for needing to replace the thyroid hormone his body cannot produce. So why do I judge myself for needing to replace the neurotransmitters that it is struggling to produce?

After a few days I felt the hint of a smile like the sunshine breaking through the clouds. In two weeks I was able to have conversations with people. In three I was able to start writing again. In five I was able to start the final edits of this book. The sun shone outside too, an eight-week heatwave, the longest in memory brought with it drought to this once muddy land.

I was home. This medicine, the right medicine, in low doses, in partnership with sunshine and swimming in the sea that nearly took me that day, reaching out to my people and walks on the beach and massage and making spirals of stones, taking flower remedies and nourishing dinners were the way back from the dark terror of my mind into my body.

The bridge back to myself that I am still walking, step by step.

And yet sometimes the waves still crash, and the sea churns and the fog falls.

But I was walking home towards myself. And it was then that the final piece fell into place, my real life medicine woman appeared, at last. She sent me a letter in the post. Courtesy of the System. No charge. No limit. She was offering a space to sort through the pieces, to stop slipping in the endless mud of the past, a chance to finally move on.

She offered me my first appointment with her.

On my birthday.

I have told you before, my life is stranger than fiction. Medicine Woman had been holding space for me all along.

MEDICINE QUESTIONS

Dr Christiane Northrup states "Disease is not created until a woman feels frustrated in her attempts to effect changes that she needs to make in her life."

How does this correspond with your own experience of illness?

In what areas of your life do you feel stuck or powerless right now?

Are you aware of where in your body your energy is stuck? Do you know what is blocking it?

How can you get yourself moving?

What words do you need to say? To who? What do you need to express?

The Feminine

What does the Feminine mean to you?

What does it look like?

Who or what represents it?

How is your definition similar or different to mine? What have I said that has changed – or clarified – your own understanding?

What has your relationship to the Feminine been over the course of your life?

How and why has it changed? What helped you to form your views?

How does the Feminine relate to the Masculine for you? Ideologically and in your own lived experience?

HEALING ARTS

Stuck

Can you describe what your current experience of feeling stuck might look or feel like using a metaphor? Does my metaphor of being stuck in the mud work for you? Or are you stuck in a cage or imprisoned? Are you submerged underwater or cornered by an enemy force? Are you abandoned in a desert without water or landlocked? Are you adrift on the waters without a way of steering your vessel? Are you frozen in a block of ice?

How can you represent this stuckness visually – can you do it through movement, by sculpting it with clay, by drawing it? Does it remind you of another time in your life?

Can you embody this feeling of stuckness literally? So if you feel stuck in ice, hold an ice cube, and watch as it transforms. If you are stuck in a ring of fire, light a bonfire or attend one. If you are stuck in sinking sand, get to the beach. See how your body physically responds to this literal embodiment of this metaphor that your mind is inhabiting. Can you see ways in which this metaphor is appearing literally in life – in the landscape, in your dreams, in the books, film or art you are drawn too?

Can you find or make yourself a magic wand to dissipate your stuckness? Are there magic words you can utter to unfreeze this stuck energy, to break the spell?

Planting Seeds of Hope

The force that through the green fuse drives the flower
Drives my green age; that blasts the roots of trees
Is my destroyer.
And I am dumb to tell the crooked rose
My youth is bent by the same wintry fever.

Dylan Thomas

What seeds can you plant to get you through the dark times? Something to watch and marvel at as it grows, something that makes visible for you the ever-unfurling process of the life-force outside of your body. You are able to witness and enjoy the flowers, perhaps the fruits, and then see how natural the process of dying back is too. If you are wanting a longer unfurling, then plant a tree. Or be more metaphorical: plant the seed of an idea in another, book yourself a healing appointment, or tickets for something you love – plant your hope in the future and dare yourself to grow towards it.

Flowers of hope. Sweet peas and cornflowers.

I bought the seeds for these a week after I couldn't even get off the floor and get dressed, I was so anxious and depressed. It was a project of hope to keep me here. It took me several more weeks to plant them. It took all my energy to plant them out. And now here they are. I pick a bunch every couple of nights and put them in a vase by my bed and go to sleep smelling their beautiful scent, and wake up to their glory each morning.

Instagram post

Cycle Charting

It is empowering to be able to witness our own progress and to track it. It gives us a sense of agency and power over our situation, as the experience of being 'in' it can be overwhelming and all consuming. The constant 'now' of illness, with seemingly little or no progress is dispiriting. Positive information bolsters our energy, our courage, our resolve to do the hard work, make the less habitual choices which support our health. Positive feedback can include photographs of ourselves – so that we can see our changes in skin, circulation, swelling, weight, hair growth, colour. They might include charting behaviour or symptoms, weighing, measuring, blood or urine tests. This helps us to assimilate the new information of our current state into our mental image of ourselves, rather than acting upon an outdated inner image or old data, which do not bear much relationship to our current reality.

Create a visual representation of the cycles of your body – your menstrual cycle, your sickness. Chart your symptoms daily. You may want to use my book *Full Circle Health* as a guide and starting point to this.

Five Minute Unblockers

Here's a little list of things you can do in five minutes to help to get yourself unstuck when you have little energy, time or space.

① Put on your favourite song, the one you need to listen to right now and move as you can – if you're bed-bound just wriggle your fingers or toes, sway your shoulders or head if you can, move your hips gently if you can. If you can stand on the floor, do, barefoot.

Close your eyes and just move in ways that feel good, starting from very small movements. You can close the door, close the curtains, listen on head phones. If you are able, sing along too.

- ◐ Clap your hands and stamp your feet, circle your hips clockwise and anticlockwise, if you're able, spin around in circles and see if that feels good.

- ◐ Use a vibrator or your fingers to explore your body and follow your pleasure.

- ◐ If there's one nearby and you're able, sit, have a go on a swing or hammock.

- ◐ Bounce on a trampoline if that's something that works for your body.

- ◐ Walk, jog or perhaps skip to the end of your road.

- ◐ Take your shoes off and walk on the sand or grass.

- ◐ Get wet! Have a shower, a bath, dip your toes in a stream, sea or fountain.

- ◐ Light a fire or a candle and focus on the flames.

- ◐ Do a clapping game with a child or good friend.

- ◐ Make a spiral in the sand if you're near a beach and then walk around it.

- ◐ Get a box of buttons or other different coloured/shaped objects (spices, beads, pens or pencils) – make a pattern by sorting them by colour or size.

- ◐ Take a line for a walk on a piece of paper – randomly doodle and then colour in or add details to the different areas.

I need...

If you're anything like me, naming and then asking for or claiming what you need is... challenging. If you are depressed, recuperating or you are measuring your energy in spoons, this exercise helps get into the habit of naming, acting on and prioritising what we need for our own wellbeing.

Take a blank page of thin card. Cut it into twelve to sixteeen small cards, all the same size. On each, in a different colour write the words: *I need...* at the top. Once you have done this on each card, either write, draw or collage images of the things that you need to support you. Possibilities might be nourishing food, a bubble bath, a walk, a massage, a swim, meeting up with a friend, a hug, a shower, ten minutes meditation, half an hour to create, to stretch your body.

Keep these beside your bed. Flick through them and pull one out each morning when you wake up and give yourself that... or ask someone else for the gift of it. Pull another one each evening.

Light Up Your Life

We're going to focus on your energy levels in this exercise. You may be familiar with the Spoon Theory[116] of energy (if not Google it and have a read). It is hugely resonant for so many chronic illness sufferers as a really valuable way of understanding and portioning out limited energetic resources. One of the hardest bits about being sick is having to learn to live on dramatically depleted energy resources. This can be deeply frustrating because our energy levels are often so out of our control, seemingly arbitrarily. But we can also acknowledge that there are things we can do to impact our energy levels: things that fill us up and things that drain us.

What in your life fills you with energy? And what drains you of energy? Be aware that certain things might feel initially energising, like coffee, alcohol or sugar, but long-term leave you feeling more depleted or in an addiction cycle? Whereas some forms of exercise may be initially draining but fill you with energy longer term.

First of all divide a piece of paper in three. Mark one side 'Fills me up', the central one 'Neutral', and the last 'Drains Me'. You may want to give each column a colour to reflect its title, so perhaps yellow for the Fills Me Up column, white for Neutral, and grey for Drains Me. Next, take a mental journey through the previous day. Put all the activities you did at home or at work into the appropriate column, remember to include hobbies, chores, exercise, caring responsibilities, self-care, spiritual practices...

On another list, you can do the same for all the foods and drinks you consumed over the course of a week.

Then using only the things that you have identified as being energising, create a visual piece – either a list in vibrant colours, or a collage or WORD + image piece, – and put it somewhere you will see it every day, perhaps in the front of your journal, beside your bed or on the fridge, as an inspiration to incorporate more of these into your daily life.

Next have a look at the tasks, activities and foods that drain you. How can you eliminate or minimise them from your daily life? Can you ask someone to do them for or with you? Can you pay someone to do them or swap them with someone? Can you set a fixed time for dealing with them, rather than them dominating your day? Can you find a more enjoyable way of doing them or a valid alternative that would be more pleasurable? Can you shift your mindset about them?

RECLAIMING

THIS IS THE TIME OF RECLAIMING

Medicine is part of our heritage as women, our history, our birthright.
Barbara Ehrenreich and Deirdre English,
Witches, Midwives and Nurses

We are the descendants of generations of women who were told that they were sinful or crazy. We are the descendants of generations of women who were not believed. We are the descendants of women who had to hide their ability to heal on pain of death.

This is the time of reclaiming.

We are reclaiming the lost Feminine and birthing it through our shame-less female bodies, into the modern world. We are reclaiming lost Feminine voices and self-expression and listening to them at last. We are reclaiming our communities as places where these values are cherished. We are reclaiming our magic.

We are reclaiming healing ritual. We are reclaiming our intuition as a valid and necessary way of knowing. We are reclaiming our connection with each other, the natural world and directly to soul and spirit. We are reclaiming a direct connection to our own life-force. We are reclaiming the wholeness of ourselves, our lightness and our dark.

We are reclaiming the traditions of our people – forgotten, punished, ignored, supplanted. And gratefully relearning the ways of other healers from those who have kept their traditions alive against all odds, through times of peril.

In this the time of the great unravelling,[117] it is time to reclaim our birth-right.

THE POWER OF BELIEF

Alice laughed. 'There's no use trying,' she said.
'One can't believe impossible things.'
'I daresay you haven't had much practice,' said the Queen. 'When I
was your age, I always did it for half-an-hour a day. Why, sometimes
I've believed as many as six impossible things before breakfast.'
Lewis Carroll, *Alice's Adventures in Wonderland*

Formerly, when religion was strong and science weak, men mistook
magic for medicine; now, when science is strong and religion weak,
men mistake medicine for magic.
Thomas S. Szasz

As women we are more exposed to non-normal experiences of consciousness through the shifts in our bodyminds: being pregnant, giving birth, breastfeeding, mothering, tending the newly born and the dying, during multiple orgasm and menstruation. These are all parts of human consciousness and physical experience that no cis male has ever experienced internally. We also share the common human experiences of sickness, ritual and ceremony, drugs and dreams. At these times our awareness of other realms of consciousness, other worlds beyond our own, other forms of conscious existence can open up to us. We see impossible things, hear voices, know what cannot be known with the waking mind: things that we or others might find disturbing, comforting or insightful.

These seem to be a universal human experience regardless of age, culture or moment in history. One that, regardless of their belief systems, people who experience them attribute meaning to and consider to be of deep importance. But this is not something our culture is really open to. There is no space for these experiences in Western medicine – they are written off as delusions, brought on by mental instability, fever or dementia, the confusion of a drug-addled brain, symptoms of illness… Meaningless.

I believe that illness makes our culture uncomfortable because it brings us to the brink of the unknown and may carry us over. It gives us *lived experience* of the wider realms of reality that patriarchy denies, because they can neither explain nor control them. Illness grants us direct engagement with the forces that *actually* control healing, bringing us out of the control of the doctor/priest puppetmasters of our culture. It takes us off the map of the patriarchy, and into the dark, from which women have been banned throughout the reign of the patriarchs. It brings us to the edge of believability, it cracks the certainty we have been assured of all our lives and pours in chaos. It makes the impossible possible, again and again, and shows us how much we don't know.

Healing holds at its heart magic. But a magic that tends to only work if we believe it.

If we believe in the power of the drug we are given, if the doctors giving them do too, test after test shows that the efficacy of the placebo effect can range from 19% up to 82%. The ability of our bodies to heal themselves is that strong.

For those who believe in the power of prayer, positive affirmations and reiki, studies prove that these have an effect.

If you trust your healing ally, if you believe in their ability to heal you, this helps their ability to heal you.

If you ask your god or goddess, if you cast a spell and you believe, your belief holds some weight.

If you place your faith in nature and the interconnectedness of all things, miracles and synchronicity often seem to occur as if by magic.

It doesn't seem to matter *what* you believe, so much as your full bodymind engagement with that belief, alongside your commitment to actively engaging with treatment.

It is vital to clarify that the power of belief doesn't mean that *anything* you believe in *actually works*, rather it means that *belief itself* has a powerful healing effect on the human body. How or why we do not yet understand. Just as it is important to remember that a medicine that has strong active properties, given in the right dose to the correct ailment, will also work the majority of the time without any form of belief. Belief is important, it seems, in activating the inner healing processes of the psyche and unconscious.

In the war of *either* psyche *or* soma, the medical profession are firmly on the side of soma, of treating the bio-mechanical body. The possibility of an equally powerful psyche, and its connection to a greater consciousness, makes medicine uncomfortable, as Dr Larry Dossey explains:

> *Although it's true that intentionality, including prayer, has been used throughout history to heal illness, this practical side is not the primary contribution of the emerging evidence. The key significance is the nonlocal nature of consciousness that is suggested by these studies. This implication dwarfs whatever pragmatic benefits these studies convey.*
>
> *Many sceptics realize what's at stake here. If only a single one of these studies is valid, then a nonlocal dimension of consciousness exists. In this case, the universe is different than we have supposed, and the game changes. Therefore, all these findings must be rejected, or the conventional, cherished views of consciousness as a completely local phenomenon will be subverted. That is why many critics seem to consider scepticism a blood sport and why they pursue a scorched-earth policy in which all studies in the field of healing are categorically condemned, often for the flimsiest reasons.[118]*

Our Western medical tradition gives short shrift to matters of belief, to the effects of consciousness on matter, or on the ability for things to transform in inexplicable manners (unless of course they were experienced by men in Biblical times). They pour scorn on synchronicities as unconnected coincidences, talk of confirmation bias, and any time something happens which is not understood, the veracity of the initial illness is put in doubt. And so women, rather than having healed themselves or having found healing elsewhere, are seen as having imagined the illness in the first place, or rather having exaggerated it, as the authorities always suspected. The term 'psychosomatic' is wheeled out and spat as a curse word of women's credulity and ability to be hoodwinked by their own weak minds, rather than an acknowledgment of the power of mind over matter, of consciousness interacting creatively with the body or of the very real physical experience of spirit or soul.

And so mainstream science seeks to annihilate or dismiss what it cannot contain within its paradigm. Even though more and more people are experiencing firsthand the ways that this paradigm simply does not fit reality. Eventually enough of us will have experienced the reality beyond the patriarchal paradigm and will compare notes. We will learn, at long last, to believe each other, believe ourselves and believe it.

Medicine Woman is leading us beyond the constraints of our cultural beliefs towards a paradigm that reflects reality as it is. Even if that makes us uncomfortable. She is guiding us towards a reality that integrates the seen and unseen, the known and unknown. A reality that asks us to trust, to have faith in what we do not yet understand, rather than dismiss it out of hand. It asks us to trust our bodyminds and their experience of reality, rather than our outdated cultural narrative.

IN MY DREAMS

For years and years, all my adult life in fact, I have been running for buses and trains in my dreams. I always thought it was just mental residue of my stressful student years commuting across London. In these dreams I was running to catch a train or bus, turning up to platforms just as they pulled away, often with my children on board.

But this past year, as my healing process has gone on, the dream changed at a significant point, and since the final part of the book came through it has stopped entirely.

On the night after I wrote the "Trauma" section, I had a dream. This time the underground train had slowed down. On it I saw myself. Reading a book. And I realised that this book was a time travel device, that it was a way of me being able to connect with other parts of myself, older and younger, outside of time. Books were my portal that I could step through and meet my timeless self and gain insight and wisdom… but most of all regain a sense of being home. This, I want to emphasise, was not just metaphorical, but literal. The girl on the train was me. I had spent my whole adult life trying to get back to her.

As I finished the last edits of the book, and realised the centrality of the psyche thread, I had a breakfast epiphany. The dreams finally made sense. I wouldn't even tell my husband the aha! moment, because I knew he, as you probably will now if I could hear you, would say, "But, of course!"

Bear with me. It took me twenty years to figure this one out, so humour me as I reveal this life-changing revelation.

Drum roll please!

The buses and trains are my metaphorical vehicles, my body.

The person trying to board them is my psyche, the part of me that identifies as me.

The train (my body) was always moving too fast (I kept myself busy all the time trying to outrun my fear, stress and anxiety brought on by not understanding my female autistic bodymind.) It never felt safe to be me, to have my psychic energy in my body in this world, and so early on I learned very effectively to separate the two. But my psyche was desperately trying to catch the train or bus: trying to reunite with my body, so that I was no longer living in a permanently dissociated state. However the trains and buses were always running to other people's timetables and schedules, they were literally being driven by someone else. Always male. The driver whose attention I was always trying to get so that he would slow down and let me on. I (being a poor runner in real life as well as my dreams!) could never quite catch them. And so there was this feeling of frustration and disappointment and missing where I was supposed to be. Again and again I missed that fucking bus. I ran whole marathons in my dreams, waking up each morning exhausted.

I don't have the dreams anymore, because after a life of running from myself, of denying my mental reality, I have finally caught up to myself. I am, more than ever before, living at my own pace. I am no longer racing to be a passenger of the patriarchy.

This running for public transport thing revealed another fascinating twist: I never was the driver in my dreams. In *The Women's Book of Dreams* which I devoured in the early stages of writing this book, I noticed that there was nearly a whole chapter on dreams about driving and cars. But no mention of buses. I put this down to it being written by a wealthy white American, about other wealthy Americans, folks who never had to use public transport, so it wasn't in their psyche, the stress of what happens if you miss the bus, literally and metaphorically. And I think this is true. But it goes deeper still. A car gives a sense of autonomy over the journey, something I have rarely felt. But in understanding my bodymind, I gained this. And so I started to drive in my dreams.

Another entirely new thing, or rather person, appeared in my dreams at the same time.

Whilst in my dreams I spend lots of time with my husband, children, old loves, father, school friends, wise women and random strangers, I could not recall ever dreaming about my mother. And suddenly, in the midst of healing my wounded Feminine, there she was too. At last.

And finally, a week before the book was finished, I saw Medicine Woman in my dreams for the first time. She was both not as I was expecting and exactly how I was. Tall, thin, wizened and wise she offered me a plate of disgusting looking plant medicines. I was too scared to try any, but got over my aversion and tried a spiralling fern shoot. She disappeared to her Temple on the cliffs, the temple I had always heard of but never knew existed, and there were all the women, gathered, fierce and strong, together.

RECLAIMING REST

'I rested,' I told her. Normally, I would have said, 'I did nothing,' but I didn't say that. I had been healing, and that's something.[119]
Firoozeh Dumas

To survive we must begin to know sacredness.
The pace which most of us live prevents this.
This Bridge Called My Back
edited by Cherrie Moraga and Gloria Anzaldua

The thing that most of us need when we are sick, that we can't get from any pharmacist or doctor is rest. Time to rest. Permission to rest. The ability to lay everything down, not against a clock, but for as long as it takes to get better.

Before Western medicine had so many medications and operations at its disposal, when the pace of life was slower, convalescence was considered a key part of healing. People were put on enforced bed rest, they stayed in convalescent homes, nursing homes, hospitals for weeks or months.[120]

Whilst the enforced nature of this was often a further way to dis-able and dis-empower many women, who had little choice about whether or not they wanted to rest or even be in these places of recuperation for extended periods, cutting them off from family and community life, we have come too far in the opposite direction, expected to work through illness and return to jobs as soon as possible.

Rest is no longer a valid option on the prescription pad – we simply don't have the time to drop everything to heal. Doing nothing is associated with laziness and a lack of productivity – both cardinal sins in the modern world.

But we must reclaim the right to rest if we are to heal.

RECLAIMING STRENGTH

How do we prepare ourselves for radical shifting? This is where women are really good. Women are used to keeping the process of life going in spite of everything – earthquakes, hurricanes, vast migrations, wars...
Virginia Sendel De Lamaitre,
Femme: Women Healing the World

Just as in *Burning Woman*, where we reclaimed what power actually is when it is inclusive of the Feminine expressions of power, so in *Medicine Woman* we reclaim what strength actually is through the experience of navigating and managing illness and disability. It is when we are most tested that we discover an inner strength we might always have doubted we had, and realise that it is very different to what we have been taught strength to be.

In the patriarchal model strength is silence – in the Feminine strength is sharing stories. In patriarchy strength is muscular strength, physical and emotional armour, in the Feminine it is the power of vulnerability. It is the inner strength to navigate the inner and outer realms of suffering, and not choose to be immune to them or unpenetrated (for in the masculine penetration is the ultimate weakness) but to subsume them into our physical and emotional selves and transform their energies.

I previously thought of myself as strong and energetic; and though I am now too, it is different, it has become a more subtle, fluid idea and embodiment of strength. There is more vulnerability now. I had to ask people for help and support in a variety of ways and aspects of my life, more so than I ever had before I was ill. This was vital, so as not to expend unnecessary energy, as when I was in the depths of illness — where I could not get out of bed and was extremely weak — I simply had no choice. Cooking, finances, where I lived, all of this changed. It taught me of my own worth and validity as a person; it showed me that I am loved and people will love me no matter if I am ill or well. I had a strong dose of activist-persona, which is great if you want to change the world but not so helpful if you're unwell and unable to help out. This meant I had to learn my 'worth' was still just the same even when I did not 'contribute' to the world. In other words, I'd been living and measuring my self-worth — and sometimes still do, this is an ongoing learning for me — by a very results-oriented mindset. It went something like: 'My worth is proportionate to my output, my actions in the world'. I knew, of course, somewhere inside me that this was not true, but I had to try to reverse the effects of such a belief and societal conditioning, I had to try turning it around.

CIARA

There is no guarantee of how much pain we will have to endure, nor for how long, when we begin the healing process. Healing requires that we find ways to navigate through painful experiences whilst staying connected to our core selves. We find ways to shed the shells, behaviours and habits that have contributed to our suffering and prevent our healing, whilst strengthening the parts of us that have become frail. As our shells crack, we begin to make contact once again with our core self, and the creative forces within.

What we feel,

This is real.

RECLAIMING HEALING COMMUNITY

Each time women gather in circles, the world heals a little more.
Unknown

We are part of the circle. When we plant, when we weave, when we write, when we give birth, when we organize, when we heal, when we do what we're afraid to do, we are not separate. We are of the world and each other, and the power within us is great, if not an invincible power. Though we can be hurt, we can heal; though each one of us can be destroyed, within us is the power of renewal.
Starhawk

Our bodies are repositories of the past – we hold history within our cells. Not just our own history, but our shared past. Just as the body remembers trauma from a car crash twenty years ago, it also remembers wars and abuse of generations past. It remembers our mother's experiences and acts as an echo chamber for our children's. It feels the stories of our sisters as its own.

When we heal within the Feminine we do not treat the body as an independent machine, but the human as one cell within a larger body: a family, a community, a shared history. Though each of our sicknesses is unique to us, and our healing must be initiated by us, it is not individual – it is a community practice. We heal together.

As humans, as women, we heal best in supportive communities – communities who will stand for us, bring soup, help care for our children, collect our medicines, listen to our fears, pay the bills we cannot, drive us to appointments, rub our shoulders, bring flowers and herbs, walk with us, watch a movie with us, pray with us and celebrate us – as we were, as we are, as we will be. Today the community is holding us, next year it will be our turn to hold another, to offer with love what she and her family needs.

Some magic is unleashed when we take our courage in our hands and name our truths within our communities, when we share our wounds and allow ourselves to be seen as vulnerable, when we dare to reach out and heal together. In these spaces our healing gives permission for others to heal. Our messiness and vulnerability give permission to others. As we grow in confidence and strength, we inspire others to do the same by our courageous example. We share the resources we have discovered, offer the support we once needed. And in doing this the medicine continues to cycle between us.

And this is what we forget in our isolation: we all hold medicine for each other. It lies hidden within our scars and the vulnerable places in our journeys. A massive part of our individual and collective healing is to share these hard-won medicines – so that they continue to work on us and on others. This is the real medicine – the collective medicine of being together on the journey – the collective remembering that in the end we are all just walking each other home.

Do you have a place of belonging (or preferably several) where you can lay down your mask for a moment, to stop hiding, to stop pretending that you can do normal… to crumble, be vulnerable, and in the midst of this to find your strength, to be accepted as you are? Is there a safe space where you can let go of old stories and find new ways to health, to share resources and support? If not, then please make this a priority in your life. This may be with friends on the ground or via email or message, a counsellor or therapist, in an online group, a red tent, a women's group, a recovery group… It needs to be a place that you can check in regularly. However you are. With people that will care enough to check in on you if they don't hear from you. And are strong enough to hold you. However you are.

I know that the initial reaching out can be hard, my love. If you have an autistic brain like mine, if you're anxious or depressed, if you can't speak or can't hear, if you are confined to bed for a hundred different reasons then you may have to find different ways of building a community, of being heard and held. For me it was the prosaic medium of a Facebook message when selective mutism meant that I could not even find the words to speak to the people I shared a house with, when I couldn't break the silence another way. The silence, whatever it is that makes you hold it, is the ice from the long winter. Reaching out to your healing allies – your doctor, your community, your nurse, the anonymous helpline, the circle, your parents or the Earth – that is spring breaking through. You can find a way, and you will.

You need a lot of support to do this work. You need to be carried on this journey sometimes, to be fed and watered as you crawl, because that's all you can do as walking is beyond your level of exhaustion. And it's up to us to carry you when that's needed. Because we who are also changing the world need carrying a lot of the time too. We can carry each other. Join together when needed if our individual energy can't do it alone – and why should we do it alone?

ROSIE

When we break our silence on the pain and shame we carry with trusted others, we put down our lonely burden. Our suffering is shared between the group. Seeds of new possibility are sown. A soul community rises up from mutual belonging and assistance. Healing moves between us, is born through us and blossoms into the world.

PICKING UP THE PIECES

There has been another meltdown. During it, the jigsaw puzzle that we have nearly finished has been broken into pieces. My eye falls on this metaphor with ironic recognition. I am too tired to yell, too empty to cry, too stubborn to put the pieces back in the box. I have invested too much time and effort in it to give up now. Instead I pull a towel off the drying rack and sit down on it on the cold bathroom floor and begin, piece by piece, to put it back together. As I work my hands begin to shake less, my breathing deepens.

Piece by piece we put our days, our love, our lives back together. Again and again. Though the possibility is always there to put the pieces back in the box and be done with it once and for all.

Most days we find a way to keep on with the puzzle we have. We know the weak spots well by now. We know that it doesn't take much to break it again. That it will break again.

Most of the time we are stuck in the details. We have poor light and have lost the lid. But still we carry on, picking and sorting, turning over the pieces in our hands, guided by some sense of the bigger picture.

We do it because we love the picture, the tiny details, the challenge of doing it, of creating meaning from chaos.

This is what we do. We are the puzzle solvers.

CHANGING THE STORY

Owning our story and loving ourselves through that process is the bravest thing that we will ever do.
Brené Brown

No matter what has happened in her life, a woman has the power to change what that experience means to her and thus change her experience, both emotionally and physically.
Therein lies her healing.
Dr Christiane Northrup,
Women's Bodies, Women's Wisdom

How are you feeling? she asks, *After the intensity of the past nine months?*
It has changed me, I reply, *I am a different person. It has broken my brain.*

Broken? she questions. *I would suggest perhaps another choice of word would be more helpful. You are not broken: you are healing.*

I am healing.

The words that we use to describe our illnesses, our bodies and ourselves shape our inner experience of their reality: words matter. The narrative structure that weaves them together – the meaning we give to these words, the relationships that they describe, the images they evoke for us matter. These words in-form our realities, our perceptions, our bodymind's internal responses.

But most of the time we do not question these narratives. We simply imagine that there is a set of facts, and that we are giving an accurate and unbiased account of them. We are unconscious storytellers of inherited truths.

The words and images we choose to define ourselves and our lives shape us. When we use them repeatedly, we become their creation. We create ourselves in their image.

In order to be able to write a new story for ourselves and for the world, in order to be able to refashion our life energy into new designs, we have to become aware of our old stories – individual and collective. We have to excavate to the founding myths: the stories that we tell ourselves and the world about who we are, how we work, why we are that way and hold them up to the light. We have to understand what symbols hold power over us, where our fear is holding our power hostage. We have to learn what it is that is disconnecting us from our life-force, and, ultimately, is making us believe in the diminished and 'sick' version of ourselves.

We inhabit an era of alternative truths. We feel – but we are told we should not. We feel what we are told is not true, what we see around us isn't real, or doesn't matter: only their script or narrative is the truth.

What we feel *is* real. What we see *does* matter.

The bodily symptoms we are experiencing are real. But perhaps their meaning is on a different level.

Our conscious, rational brains have been so conditioned to the superficial stories and symbols of our culture that it is only our unconscious that can jolt us from the communal daze of patriarchy – through dreams and hallucinations to see what lies beneath.

Healing often requires re-storing our self-belief, our values, what life means to us and our relationship with it. It means *re-storying* ourselves: reclaiming the language of our bodies, the meaning that we attribute to them and our right to define them. It requires the sharing of our personal stories of sickness and healing with those who can fully witness their value and empathise with our pain. It starts when we take the lead in our own definition – understanding ourselves through the lens of our conditions whilst paradoxically knowing ourselves as much more than just our medical labels. It continues apace when we reclaim the narrative of our lives. In the words of esteemed Jungian analyst, Marion Woodman, "To hear the Feminine we have to dare to open our receptors to old words with new meanings."[121]

Learning to tell the story of who we are, and how we got here is a vital part of the healing process. Through so-called narrative medicine[122], we can begin to understand the purpose of our stories, and how they are interwoven with the stories of our families and others like us. In short, we learn to belong again to ourselves. To our communities. To the world. In healthy ways. We can find our tribes and build new gathering places. Together we can co-author a new story of what it means to be human. Discovering that we hold some power to influence the ending is deeply empowering. In contrast to the patriarchal, scientific model which asserts that we are damaged individuals who are powerless to effect change, unless we are Establishment experts or heroes.

Rather than victims of a story that we had no part in penning, in narrative medicine we take an active role. Rather than victims of our illness, we engage with it directly: we change what we can, in order to prioritise our own wellbeing, and centre our own reality.

As women, as a culture, we have to recognise that the fairy tale of happily-ever-after, of being scared of the witch in the forest, of staying on the well-lit path and out of the dark is a myth, not a blueprint for reality. We have been taught to exchange every part of our power for the dream of the handsome man who will save us, the castle in the clouds – the towering phallus of power and prestige leading up into the light. Our ego has been trained for this longing since childhood. Our persona is carefully polished and honed to achieve this. But the dark Feminine soul knows she needs to sink deep to find her power. She knows she needs to unravel the wool and spin a new cloth from the stories she has found in her own soul. The body knows what it knows. It has been waiting for us to stop dreaming of castles in the air and start listening to its wisdom: inhabiting it as the sacred space it is.

Many traditional forms of medicine, from Native American, to Maori[123] and Aboriginal[124] healers, and within Western European culture, Jungian therapists, family constellation and art therapists use narrative, myth, story and imagery to help the sick person understand their suffering in terms of the soul's language of imagery, but also as a way of integrating their experiences with those of their ancestors and culture. Through this form of healing the patient becomes aware of many other myths beyond the dominant white patriarchal ones and many other roles and identities which may fit them better. They rediscover a heritage which reflects and empowers them. They find a new home and identity for their psyches both in their own bodies, communities and in the world at large.

Whatever culture we come from we can learn from this deeply

human way of healing: the power of story. We humans are meaning-makers. And sickness is no exception to this deep need to make sense of our experiences. Consciously re-storying our existence lies at the heart of healing. We need to take our focus from the compulsion of fixing our bodies, and extend it to the ultimately more necessary project of integrating our souls and accepting our bodies in their diversity.

We can see powerful examples of this in the work of many well-known female creatives: Frida Kahlo, Audre Lorde, Virginia Woolf, Sylvia Plath, Susan Sontag and Eve Ensler are just some who have sought to gain self-understanding, self-expression and healing through their courageous acts of giving voice to their sickness, in a culture that would have preferred that they remain silent. As Virginia Woolf says, in *On Being Ill*:

> *Considering how common illness is, how tremendous the spiritual change that it brings, how astonishing, when the lights of health go down, the undiscovered countries that are then disclosed, what wastes and deserts of the soul a slight attack of influenza brings to light [...] what ancient and obdurate oaks are uprooted in us in the act of sickness, how we go down into the pit of death and feel the waters of annihilation close above our heads and wake thinking to find ourselves in the presence of the angels [...] it becomes strange indeed that illness has not taken its place with love, battle, and jealousy among the prime themes of literature.*

It is up to each of us to help to normalise sickness through sharing our stories, and to contribute to helping to make the healing journey more meaningful. We can do this by making our stories less insular, less of a monologue, by seeing the similarities first between ourselves and others in our communities, and then the connections between our own suffering and the imbalance in the world beyond us. This act of re-storying our experiences with our own bodies and voices is not just of benefit to us individually. One of the most challenging aspects of Western industrial medicine is the intense focus on individual therapies and diagnostic language all of which can leave us feeling alienated, scared, alone and rejected from our peers, community and selves.

The most definitive difference between an alternative approach to health and Western medical treatment is the belief that there is a mental and emotional root to all physical ailments. Where Western medicine asserts that illness is meaningless, simply the dysfunction of a machine that needs repairing, alternative medicine approaches believe that illness and the process of healing from it are profoundly meaningful, that consciousness is at the root of both the physical and emotional issues, both as source and fount of healing potential.

As we begin to move into the metaphorical, we enter a new realm where meaning is as important as matter and where matter is informed by meaning. Consciousness, attention and interpretation hold a transformative power in this realm: one that can in-form, and ultimately shift the trajectory of our worldly experiences. We reclaim 'psychosomatic' as a term of power.

It can be really hard to understand the metaphorical journey of sickness and healing when you are feeling isolated and fully engaged with the pain and misery of living it. But being able to share the experience and being able to access the experiences of others, be it through art or words or group meetings, helps to ensoul and humanise the process. Allowing time and space to reflect on and integrate your experience as you heal can prevent you from re-walking the same path again and again.

One of the shifts that may come from the creative and narrative approach to healing is a change in our relationship with our illness. In scientific medicine a tumour or rash tends to be treated as an invasive entity, influenza nothing more than the symptoms of a viral infection. Whereas when we begin to look symbolically or metaphorically at them, when we begin to understand them not just as annoyances to be gotten rid of, but as communications from our body, as our body's intelligent and creative responses to something, we in turn feel able to engage creatively with them. To enter into dialogue, rather than feel victimised by them.

Though it may feel a little strange at first, to become acquainted with a part or our bodies or a ball of cells, may I gently suggest that you find a way to engage with the spirit or soul of the illness, to inquire as to why it came to you, what its purpose is, what it is trying to teach or show you, what it is trying to move you away from or towards.[125] We may begin to see that each symptom has its own personality, identity, purpose or lesson.[126]

This narrative engagement might take place in your imagination, in your dreams, out loud alone or with a friend or therapist, in your journal, on canvas, in a meditation or in letters. As we begin to enter this realm of creative engagement with ourselves, our lives and our illness, we enter a metaphysical realm in which the physical, mental and energetic are more closely connected than Western culture allows for. We begin to notice the metaphorical reality that we inhabit, and the intelligence that imbues it. We awaken to the multiplicity of many conscious entities and their story arcs that influence each other in previously unseen ways within our bodyminds and lives. We understand on an experiential level our interrelatedness.

The use of symbolic or ritual actions is a vital part of this process. We use our body, our hands, feet, arms, legs, hips and chest, to integrate our psychological experience, journeying with our body what our mind is journeying, and vice versa, yoking the experience of the two together, and allowing each to provide its own insight and intelligence.

I invite you to look for the symbolic and embrace it on your healing journey. Find outer expressions of the inner metaphors you have been discovering: knit a scarf as your bones knit together, balance rocks as you learn to find inner balance, tidy your home as you sort through the old parts of your psyche, create a patchwork made of old clothes as you piece together the parts of yourself that have been lost, embark on a challenging physical adventure as you navigate the internal terrain of grief.

Again, I caution that this approach is not used *instead* of focusing on healing the body, but as a way of engaging all of your intelligences in order to heal more thoroughly. Small shifts in the fabric of our consciousness can make big changes within our bodyminds. Working at this level helps us to experience a sense of co-creation and a greater power. The healing arts exercises in this book have been a way of helping you engage in small supported steps with this process. This book itself is doing the same. The resources section is packed with more support.

Together we are untangling the threads of our sickness.

Together we are rewriting the story of what it means to be human and what it means to heal.

WHAT'S RIGHT WITH ME?

It is no measure of health to be well-adjusted to a profoundly sick society.
Krishnamurti

I have spent a lifetime absorbing all the things that our culture believed was wrong with me because my body is female, because I express emotions fully, because I embody the Feminine.

I have spent half a lifetime writing lists of what is wrong with me: unpicking my symptoms, fixating on my imperfections, apologising for my flaws, trying to figure it all out alone.

I have spent decades wondering why I did not fit in, why I was so weird, as though that were a bad thing.

Now I wonder if my not fitting in were actually a sign of health, not sickness. If not fitting in is actually what may save me. Because I can see the reality I inhabit more clearly, because I do not, cannot, properly fit into it.

I have spent so many years cursing my weirdness, my not-normalness, that I never realised what a precious gift it was. It is. My consciousness is rich and diverse. She is multifaceted and shining, she is chameleon-like and chaotic, she is dark and murky, she is full of bone-shaking fear. But she is mine. She is filled with wild yeast and rises within me in bubbles of bliss.

I have spent so much of my time trying to do things right (according to the rules of others), rather than do them well, rather than doing what I wanted in my way.

I have spent so much of my energy trying to repress or control the life-force that came through my body, shutting down the voice that came through it, because I was too scared of what would happen when it emerged into the world. I was too scared of what happens to women like me. Too scared of what is done to our bodies.

I was so scared that I shut down. And this powerful energy played havoc within me instead.

But this life-force, She, is needing to emerge, her ways are longing to be born, heard, seen. The life-force belongs here, through us. That is our only job, our only role here. This man-made world, this masculine-dominated culture tells us it's wrong, we're wrong. But it's not, it's not. It is so desperately needed.

It is time to change the story. To stop defining myself by what I am not.

My body has been a power cell for the patriarchy, my mind a super computer.

I am logging off. I'm going to be a conductor for the Feminine.

I am going to start writing lists of my capabilities, gifts, abilities and wild mysteries, I am going to focus on harnessing the magic within me.

Instead of trying to fix myself, or fix the world, I am freeing myself from the confines of trying to belong to a broken world.

Instead of begging for their medicine, begging for their concern, begging to be heard, to be taken seriously, I will take my own medicine and offer it widely.

Instead of trying to fit myself to the vision and expectations the world holds for me, I will make my own and share it.

Instead of accepting my inferiority I will assert my rights. Instead of quietening my voice so as not to be any trouble, I will raise it.

Instead of putting everyone else first, instead of being an after-thought, I will be my own first priority. I will make space for myself.

Rather than collapsing inwards in fear and silence, I reach out to my sisters and brothers, my medicine people, my circles of support. There is no shame in my suffering.

My willingness to share my pain is my medicine. It opens the possibility of healing, not only to myself, but to all those who I am in community with.

My commitment to tending myself, to speaking my messy truth, to sharing my vulnerability, to receiving support are a gift and a blessing.

This is my body.
This is my life.
This space I inhabit is my territory.
This energy is mine.
This power is mine.
For years I gave myself away, apologising in the process.

I burned my energy unthinkingly,
Wasted it, squandered it,
I threw good after bad.
For years I ran on empty
Feeling it was all I deserved.
Only keeping the dregs for myself.
But now I am reclaiming it.
I will nurture it for the gift it is.
I give thanks for my unique consciousness
I am deeply grateful for this body.
And so I embark on the path less travelled.
All around me sick women are doing the same.
Something is shifting within us. Something bigger than us as individuals.
Some point to Mayan prophecies or the shift in the stars
A new astrological age,
Our consciousness rising to higher frequencies.
Some only see the collapse of patriarchy,
And believe the foretold end is nigh.
But we can feel Her rising within us.
We can see our sisters rising around us.
The Feminine is being reborn in us, through us.
The Feminine is rising
Through our exhausted broken bodies…
She is rising.
The scales are being balanced once more.
We are healing ourselves, healing the Earth.
We are healing.
Together.
At last.

MEDICINE QUESTIONS

Belief

What does 'being believed' or 'being taken seriously' mean to you?

Do you believe yourself? What has shaken your self-belief in the past?

How do you respond if people do not believe you?

How easy or hard do you find it to argue against those you disagree with and state what you believe?

What do you believe in, and why?

HEALING ARTS

Health Check: Part Two

Remember the table of symptoms you created at the end of the "Symptoms: What's Wrong?" chapter? Now is the time to move to the possible inner meaning of them. It is vital to address our physical symptoms with a respected healing ally, to take them seriously in their physical manifestation first and foremost. But in order to heal deeply, it is useful to look at why, on an energetic level, these symptoms emerged and pay attention to them as messengers.

Take your chart of symptoms and a book such as *You Can Heal Your Life; Eastern Body, Western Mind; Women's Bodies, Women's Wisdom* or *The Secret Language of your Body*. For a simplified online version of Louise L. Hay's chart from *You Can Heal Your Life* see tinyurl.com/haysymptoms5

Each of these books has a fascinating chart of the possible psychological and energetic meanings of symptoms, including the chakras that they are related to and the possible emotional blockages that they are communicating, as well as suggested ways to shift them.

So, take your table, and if you need more room then tape another sheet of paper onto the side. Next to each of your symptoms fill out the information on the following page:

ENERGY/BODY SYSTEM AFFECTED	
MESSAGE	
POSSIBLE SOURCE	
POSSIBLE WAY TO HEAL	

Shedding the Shell

Find, paint or collage a shell that represents your transformation at this time. If you live near a beach or can visit one, go and find one for yourself that feels representative of your experience. Or you might choose to look online or in shops for a shell, or shell image. You might choose to wear it, or keep it on your altar space. Can you write about what this experience of 'shedding your shell' looks like?

Or perhaps shells are not your thing. Maybe a different natural metaphor feels more appropriate to you – is it the shedding of leaves in the autumn, pruning back last year's growth on trees or bushes, a snake shedding its skin or an animal moulting for summer? Find an image or object that represents this for you.

The Birth of a New Self

After you have grieved your self that is passing, how can you welcome the self that is emerging? What would feel good to celebrate her? Perhaps you would like to have a special ceremony or meal. You might anoint your body with scented oil or water. You may have a beautiful photograph taken. You might make or buy a new piece of clothing or accessory that marks this new identity: a piece of jewellery, a tattoo, a beautifully carved walking stick, a decorated wheelchair, a wig, a softly knitted scarf, a precious medicine pouch to carry your medications, a warm nurturing wrap to keep your womb and kidneys cosy, a beautiful patchwork blanket… You may choose a new spiritual name, or spirit guide animal or symbol. You may design a nurturing new daily ritual or routine. Is there anyone you want to invite to share this experience with you?

Joy Pockets

In the midst of our suffering, we can begin to overlook all the things we love, the little things that make life worthwhile. Many therapists recommend cultivating a daily gratitude practice, so that noticing the good in your life becomes an ingrained habit. I call this practice 'joy pockets'. Some days it is a mental list as I fall asleep, sometimes it is a list I write down and share on social media and invite others to share their gratitudes, other days it is the practice of noticing with my camera in hand, taking a snap of a little joy. Joys can be big or small: a beautiful flower in an unexpected place, the safe birth of a baby, the scent of rain on hot tarmac, witnessing or receiving a small kindness, the bus coming on time, the juiciness of a ripe strawberry, a parking space when you need one, the patterns in the clouds...

Sharing Gratitude

When we are sick many folks do a lot to help us. And, let's be honest, we can be bloody hard to deal with when we are in pain, depressed, angry and sad.

A really important part of the healing process is giving back to those who have supported us in our tough times, especially if we were unable to do so at the time (though a thank you to our carers in the midst of our suffering always goes a long way).

Most people who work in the frontline of healing are over-worked and under-appreciated. They show up for strangers in middle-of-the-night shifts, on holidays, whatever is going on in their own private lives.

They showed up for us and helped us when we needed them most. They do this work because it matters to them. They work in a System that does not value them. So tell them what a difference they have made in your life. Share your gratitude for their skills, care and dedication. Perhaps you can write a card, letter or email to each of the individuals who has helped care for you. Let them know what it was that you valued. Buy or pick them a bunch of flowers. Share a piece of your art or writing with them. Bake or buy them cookies or a cake. Throw a party for them. Phone them up or call in to see them. If they work for a hospital or charity that accepts contributions then why not give financially or volunteer, or hold a fundraising event for them. And pay it forward in their names – if they work privately, recommend them to friends and colleagues so that they have new clients. Pick up a handful of their business cards and carry them in your wallet to hand out. If they work in the public system get friends to ask to be referred to them. Keep the healing circle going, and use a portion of your life-energy to support those who give so much for others and who carry the healing flame through these dark times.

Creating Healing Community

Do you have a healing community? What role have relationships and community had in your healing/recovery so far? What does it look like and how does it help?

What are you still longing for?

How can you build your community of medicine women?

Who do you know in real life who has the same condition or is at the same stage of healing from a chronic illness? Who do you know of that is a few steps ahead? Can you make some time to meet up to talk together, perhaps over a coffee, via Skype or on a walk? Are there any local support groups for this in your area? How can you find out about what might be available? Check message boards in local doctors' surgeries, community centres, mental health centres, ask your doctor, healing ally or friends.

Where have you seen or experienced communities like this? Can you draw or write down your vision? You might want to start this as a vision board. Or you might want to create it in reality – write an invitation, create a poster, organise an event, a Facebook group...

I cordially invite you to join me and the community of women reading this book over on the "Medicine Woman – a book by Lucy H. Pearce" Facebook group.

What's Right with You?

Write or draw a list of what's right with you – all your wonderful skills and abilities, the things your bodymind is good at, the ways they work beautifully, all you are grateful to be able to do. Perhaps add doodles, illustrations or collage photographs of special bodily experiences – swimming in the ocean, eating your favourite food, skiing, dancing, hugging someone you love, with something you're proud of creating...

RENAISSANCE

A NEW NORMAL

As you move through these changing times [...] be easy on yourself and be easy on one another. You are at the beginning of something new. You are learning a new way of being.
Message from the
Council of Thirteen Indigenous Grandmothers

When we are sick, depressed, traumatised, grieving or in shock we often long to get back to normal, to return, as quickly as possible, to the way things were before. We long for solid ground. For the monotony of the mundane, the sweet blessings of the everyday, the soothing balm of habit, the lack of drama, the return of energy and vitality, for the rewards of busyness and accomplishment. We yearn for doing, not feeling.

Most of all we long to feel safe again. To feel calm and whole and good. To be independent rather than reliant on the mercies of others. To trust our bodies again. To believe that the world and its people are familiar and friendly. To believe in a loving divine power and a benevolent universe. To know that we are, as we used to believe, in control of our own destinies, rather than passengers on a cruel and stomach-churning rollercoaster ride that we didn't ask to get on... and we can't get off.

And so we rush back to normal as quickly as possible. For our own sakes. And the sakes of those we love. So that sickness is a memory, a fading bad dream.

We try to put on our old lives, but like a sweater that has shrunk in the wash it no longer fits us: the arms are too short, and it no longer covers our bellies. It is, perhaps, only then that we accept the enormity of the transformation we have undergone. Trying to fit back into our

257

old selves is like a butterfly trying to get back into its cocoon.

Coming back to life requires that you come out as who you are now – with your changes, differences, limitations and learnings. It may include a new physical appearance, new clothes or hair, a new way of getting about, new social circles, a new home or occupation. It will almost definitely require a new way of living – new eating regimes, exercise, medication, appointments, and a treasuring of your more limited energy.

But usually we find this out the hard way.

When we try to become who we once were. And fail. Our bodyminds relapse, we collapse exhausted in a puddle of hot tears, the rashes and fevers and aches and anxiety return. And once again we dive for our familiar crutches. Only to find that they can no longer take our full weight.

Or if we do manage it, so-called normal feels false, like going through the motions.

Because it is.

Because everything that was 'us' before has been thrown up in the air, broken into a million pieces. We cannot force normal... not for long anyway without further disintegration down the line.

Sickness isn't a clock watcher. It doesn't respect timetables, appointments, work days, sick leave limitations, religious holidays, the patience levels of our carers, the limits of our financial resources, our courage, our reservations ... it just keeps on going... until you surrender yourself fully. Until you find the medicine that works. And you keep on taking it. Until you can find the strength to eliminate what is making you sick. Until you let go of getting back to normal.

Because the truth that you sense is in fact the reality that everyone including you is in denial of: old normal doesn't exist anymore. It is the discarded snail shell, one size too small. It is the snake skin rolling in the wind, the dry chrysalis hanging from the branch.

With great irony we make ourselves sick, trying to get back to normal. Trying to be better.

We must embrace a new normal.

And when we finally accept this new normal as our own, when we acknowledge that everything has changed. Internally. Externally... the paradox emerges: we can also see how much everything has stayed the same.

The threads of the old run through this new reality in small ways and big… the comfort blanket of your old reality is here after all, just freshly washed in the laundry of life by Medicine Woman. The stains and daily grime washed out, a ragged bit trimmed off there, the hole stitched up, a different smell… same, same but different.

BETWEEN TWO WORLDS

We sense that 'normal' isn't coming back, that we are being born into a new normal: a new kind of society, a new relationship to the earth, a new experience of being human.
Charles Eisenstein

We live at this time between two worlds. Between the land of sickness, and of healing. Between the realm of patriarchal medicine, and the realm of Medicine Woman. On a personal scale. On a global level. But many – most even – still cannot sense or see or experience the 'world coming': they are totally invested in the old world, totally immersed in sustaining what has been, in defending and maintaining the old stories.

Western medicine works extremely well within its parameters and understanding of reality: the masculine worldview and male bodies; the non-gendered mechanics of the human body and physical trauma, and infectious disease; the stable industrial world of the nineteenth and twentieth centuries. But its inability to understand the emergent paradigm – the Feminine soul as it emerges through the female bodymind; the globalised world culture; an environment in flux; complex organic systems; a spiritual revolution – are what now make it potentially impotent or even dangerous. For that we need something else. Something we *can* believe in. Something that believes us as women and understands how our bio-energetic systems actually work. Something that doesn't discredit or deny our complex experiences of reality. Something that can treat bodymind and soul.

We are moving beyond either/or, not backwards into less knowing, but forwards into deeper, more complete ways of knowing. Our intention: to combine the achievements of Western heroic medicine with intuitive knowing and ancient ways of Feminine healing; a form of healing that combines the best of the healing arts with the healing sciences.

Though our souls may be longing for Medicine Woman, and though we may be actively trying to seek out her emissaries in the real world, still our bodies inhabit the old world. Our options may be severely limited by geography or money. We discover that we need to get a diagnosis from a medical doctor and submit to invasive (and often inconclusive) tests in order to access health insurance payments for our treatments, for sick leave, government support services and welfare payments. We need to fill out endless forms and seek out financial and social supports in a culture that has been gutted by capitalism.

For now, in every place where the System touches our lives, our reality must be approved and signed off on. So we are forced – if we have jobs, schooling, financial support, if we parent or access many community services – to continue to submit our bodies and minds to assessment and diagnosis by Western medicine that we understand to be lacking. Otherwise we are on our own. No other diagnoses or expertise will be acknowledged or accepted. If children or certain government agencies are involved, avoiding Western doctors can potentially be seen as irresponsible, abusive or even criminal.

For now, there are no acceptable alternatives to the System. Unless you live fully outside of it – which the majority of us can't and don't – Western medicine is enforced.

As a woman committed to her own healing, in her own way, you may well be seen as crazy by those who still adhere to the absolute truths of patriarchy. Because patriarchal institutions have for so long claimed dominion over our bodies, over the definition of health and sole authority to practice medicine, a woman learning to take ownership of her body, to claim personal authority, spiritual authority for herself may be perceived as cranky, difficult or even dangerous. To reject the rules is to reject the System. To reject the System is deemed unacceptable.

And so whilst we are building the new we must continue to learn to navigate the System wisely, with minimal damage to ourselves. We must band together and learn from those who have walked this path before us as to what to expect and how to find the best people and procedures it has to offer. We must teach each other who and what it is safe to trust. We must know our rights, insist upon consent-based care at all times. We must flag up the System's failings and abuses and stand together to expose them.

When we are stuck in the old world, it is up to us to build new ways.

We need new stories about what it means to be sick. What it means to heal.

For a long time in our culture, we have locked sickness up, hidden it away, in homes and institutions, in hospitals and asylums. The time has come to integrate its reality into our humanity – to accept it as part of ourselves, part of a valid expression and experience of humanity, to broaden the very narrow definition of who gets to be human – what normal looks like and sounds like. Sick people need their communities, even more than the well. They need to be connected to nature and life… just as they need also to rest and retreat. But first and foremost they need to feel human. To feel loved. To be cared for and about. And as more and more of us become sick – rather than shutting us away and pushing us away because we don't do normal so well, we need to adapt what normal is. If sickness is something that almost every human will experience at some point in their lives, if chronic sickness is something that even more of us will experience than ever before, there is no better time to create the sort of healthcare that we would like to experience at our most vulnerable, rather than the sort we will do anything to avoid at all costs.

Imagine if healthcare were integrated into our lives and communities, if it was something we looked forward to engaging with. Imagine the potential of that.

Imagine if our bodyminds were something we were excited, curious and engaged with as they developed and changed, rather than avoided or scared of.

Imagine if we embraced the full range of our conscious experience rather than just hid in one tiny part of the spectrum.

Imagine if we stopped being scared of ourselves, each other and the world, and started really living.

Imagine.

WRITING NEW NARRATIVES

One thing's for sure… if any one of us unleashes our creativity,
our world will split open. We'll find unprecedented ways of solving
problems and expressing our souls, and our lives
will be forever changed.[127]
Martha Beck

You are not broken,
You are healing.
You are not cursed by your illness,
You are blessed.
You are not alone,
We are in this together.

To heal is to be a conscientious objector to the culture of war we have inhabited as normality. To heal is to risk moving closer to death and return bringing back more life-force to our planet and deepen our understanding of our interconnections. To heal requires that we inhabit the Feminine more fully and reject the divine right of toxic masculinity to dominate.

To focus on personal healing in our culture is an act of powerful, political rebellion. It is an act of spiritual revolution. It is also a profound act of service – one which will ripple up and down your family lineage, out into your community and the world beyond you. To insist on healing for all peoples in this time is scary. But it is needed.

We are learning through our personal healing journeys that we have the power to change first our own embodied experiences and inner worlds. But what might transformation look like on a systemic level?

It looks like pushing for and supporting greater research into women's health. It looks like paying nurses and carers (the majority of whom are women) fairly for their work, and properly valuing their contribution to healing. It looks like recruiting doctors not just based on academic grades but also compassion and a caring manner. It looks like voting for politicians who are committed to investing in healthcare for all. It looks like standing for election, training as healers ourselves, so that we are embodying our understanding within the System, and co-creating new realities.

It looks like diverse and new ways of healing. Taking much of health-care out of hospitals and back out into the world – into gardens and forests and farms and our homes. Taking the pharmaceutical medicines we need, but also being open to the healing that comes from herbs and hands and movement and sound and colour. It looks like respecting, learning from and integrating other traditional methods of healing. It looks like finding and supporting healing allies who work in support of the Feminine: integrative medicine, functional medicine, community medicine… and reporting those who abuse their positions of authority whatever healing discipline they practise.

It looks like the current model and standard of care that teens with Type 1 diabetes get where we live: free medications for life for ailments connected to their condition, free and regular check ups with a personal team of medical professionals including a consultant, specialist nurse team and dietician. Well-funded international research contributing directly to greater understanding of the condition and patient care, feeding directly into a rapid advance in technology for artificially managing and replacing the function of the affected organ. Parent and child education programs in a non-medical setting, run by experts, in all aspects of management of the condition, self-care, diet and general health. Regular social activities to promote friendship and support amongst peers with the condition, including an educational element – cooking together, shopping together, eating together, playing together. Adventure weekends with full medical support so that teens can experience freedom in a safe place, try new physical activities and families can have respite from the demands of full-time caring. Family weekends away so that siblings can meet other siblings in the same situation, parents can meet other parents, and all can relax in a place that caters for their needs as standard. A dedicated nurse line to help carers manage the condition at home and advise when hospitalisation is needed. A medical system supported by a strong charitable body, staffed by professionally and personally dedicated individuals who are passionate about what they do and who see the person ahead of the condition.

It looks like the sort of project that my grandmother was involved in eighty years ago: The Pioneer Health Centre in Peckham, credited as being an inspiration for the NHS. Built in one of the poorer areas of London by a visionary pair of doctors, its approach to health was revolutionary then. And would still be today. It was centred around community health and was housed in a massive purpose-built space which included sports facilities, meeting rooms, childcare, a canteen, dance hall and the freedom for all members to engage with and organise the activities they wanted. Regular health check-ups were standard and medical care given as needed, before illness became chronic or intractable. It looked like eating and dancing and playing together. With a focus on family and community as the places where health is fostered. Health that was built around and woven through every aspect of daily life. A vision of health that prioritised the freedom of physical and energetic expression. For an affordable monthly subscription. If this description inspires you, please take twenty minutes out of your life to watch this video: tiny.cc/peckham See how dated the world looks, this pre-Second World War world, but how modern the vision.

And this is just one possibility. One vision. There are millions of ways to heal.

There are millions of souls that are already dedicated to pioneering visions of what health could be: doctors charging monthly fees so that their patients can come and see them as often as they want, not just when they are badly sick. Doctors who are training in complementary approaches: acupuncture, herbalism, chiropractic, homeopathy in order to be able to offer more in the way of healing. Death doulas and hospices providing caring homes from home with pain relief for gentle dying. Those campaigning for medicinal cannabis to be available on prescription, and for MDMA to be a valid way of treating trauma. Healers and volunteers going into hospitals to make art, tell stories, plant seeds, hold premature babies...

The lie we have been sold for far too long is that there is only one way to heal.

BRAVE WORK

We all begin the process before we are ready, before we are strong enough, before we know enough [...] We respond before we know how to speak the language, before we know all the answers, and before we know exactly to whom we are speaking.
Clarissa Pinkola Estés, *Women Who Run With the Wolves*

It is a fierce blessing to be alive right now in these times. To be living through this era of cultural and individual transformation. One that takes all our courage and determination, to live through the releasing of our communal fears and walk through the underworld to the other side, to create a new way of living.

This is brave work. For when we break with the causes of our sickness, the philosophical and energetic roots of it, we are breaking conceptually with the mindset that has defined and sustained us, with the unwritten agreements of the tribe that we were born into. We are converting from the religion of our birth, rescinding our nationality and possibly leaving our friends and family behind in that world. It feels big, scary and very daunting. And so we may try to make compromises, take half measures. We dip our toe into the new and go running back to the old for comfort, to remember who we were before.

But the old causes a flare up, and we feel trapped between a world that makes us sick, and another world so shaking and shimmering in its newness, one that we have been told to doubt and scorn all our lives. We can keep approval, ease and comfort by rejecting it, and keep our sickness too... or we can branch out, step into the new risking rejection, judgement, scorn, and possible greater health.

What a choice!

And so most of us follow the path more travelled, the one which comes with societal approval, if not necessarily relief. We take the pills and swallow them down. We have the operation. And if there are no pills, no operation, we take their word for it that nothing can be done. And we suffer in silence as we were taught.

But Medicine Woman is showing us another way. She is calling us back to life through our bodies and minds. She is calling us to healing.

She is starting a paradigm shift from within, asking us to embody our knowing. She is calling us to make our sickness visible, our suffering public. She is asking that we step out in ourselves, not as victims, not to get attention or sympathy but to say,

Stop, this is real.

This is what is happening. This is who I am. This is my lived reality. I will not hide my suffering to make life easier for you.

This is my life, my world too. It is messy, complex, ever-changing. I will not apologise for myself being less than perfect. I come as I am, I offer what I can. I am part of your community. And you are a deeply valued part of mine.

This is a vital transformation for me, and I am not ashamed.

It is time to say, in our millions,

This world, this System, is not working for me as it is now.

It is making us sick.

It is time to change.

Today it may be me, tomorrow it may be you. We stand together, whatever life may bring, whatever reality we find ourselves embodying. We put ourselves first. We share the burden of sickness, we share the joy of living.

EMBODYING OUR HEALING

I have heard it said that illness is an attempt to escape the truth. I suspect it is actually an attempt to embody the whole truth, to remember all of ourselves.
Kat Duff, *The Alchemy of Illness*

As Women Healing we are being forced to actively question and overthrow the Western lifestyle from the inside out. We're having to re-vision our working practices, diet, levels of stress and overwhelm, acceptable amounts of sleep and rest, relationship and family dynamics. We are having to build new ways of making health, new means of support, new ways of living and working on the hoof: the healing women of our world are creating a new health-giving culture by necessity.

We're not just dreaming up utopian ideas or guided by wishful thinking. We are embodying our healing, urgently, as if our lives depended on it. Because they do. It seems that the stakes needed to be this high for us to finally take action. We are grounding a new conscious awareness of what it means to be human in our Earth-bound bodies after millennia of projecting ourselves into the future, focusing on the salvation of our souls in worlds yet to come, relying on someone else to save our bodies.

We are no longer lost in the darkness of the trauma that we cannot change. We are no longer powerless. We are here, together, now, rooted in these bodies, on this Earth.

We are capable of healing. We are worthy of healing.

The power to do so is pouring through our bodies.

And we are realising (finally) that the System is not (yet) an independent entity. It is still, (just) run by humans. And is supposed to be serving humans. All humans. This is our moment, before it becomes more automated, before it is any further out of our hands. Once we have learned how to reclaim our own individual power, we can join together to collectively reclaim the System and make it work for us. But it has to work for all of us. Not just white or rich or male. Our survival as a species and individuals depends on this.

We find ourselves in the privileged but daunting position of co-creating the world we have been waiting for. A more nurturing culture. One where child and domestic care is better shared, one stripped of harmful chemicals, where holistic healing works alongside allopathic medicine, where sensitivity is not ignored, where hormones and natural cycles are better understood. A culture where health-making is prioritised and the diversity of humanity is embraced.

We are not starting from scratch. All around you, in your community, in the world, you will see folks already working hard for this. Folks pulling together to make a change – inside the System, at grass roots level, in their homes. We just have to join the dots, make the connections between these individual cells of healing, into a more coherent web that can hold us all, so that when patriarchy finally crashes down, there is something to catch us.

A FLOURISHING OF THE FEMININE

The 'damaged' woman is not damaged at all – she is wounded, and in channelling and healing her wounds, she becomes the source of incredible energy, the site of unbelievable potential for abundance and change. She possesses the power to use her wounds for the greater good and her highest good.[128]
Shahida Arabi

This is the first time that the Feminine has been embodied by women on such a mass global scale, the first time that Feminine energy has poured through so many female bodies. It is truly a collective awakening. Can you feel the energy that has been feeding your sickness, feeding the patriarchy, feeding the System, feeding everyone except yourself… can you feel it unfurling? Can you feel your power?

This is the first time in the history of humanity that technology has been able to support and connect the revolution throughout communities and around the globe. The first time enough women are well enough nourished, freed from domesticity and enforced childbirth enough to be able to focus on their greater wellbeing. The first time enough of us have access to the resources we need to help us to heal. The first time enough of us are able to read and write. The first time we are able to transcend the limits of state and language to create a global vision of healing. The first time such an array of healing modalities have been available for so many.

We are shifting the old, healing the past, in our bodies, through our bodies. We are connecting to our bioenergetic realities: connecting to our cycles of being and harnessing the power of the life-force. We are using technology to support and enhance this. Millions upon millions of women are for the first time giving free expression to their spiritual, emotional, creative and sexual selves and making themselves visible. We are creating our vision for ourselves and our cultures. We are healing ourselves, and through ourselves we are healing the world. Body by body, system by system.

We may have feared that illness had stolen our lives from us, making them meaningless. But the healing journey offers us the most meaningful experience of our lives, one we will never forget. One that will shape us. One that will turn our understanding of ourselves inside out. One that will transform our experience of what it means to be human, what it means to be alive.

The healing is coming through us, the healing is in us. We are the crucibles for it.

THE RISE OF THE NEW HEALERS

The shaman must become sick to understand sickness. When the shaman overcomes her or his own sickness she will hold the cure to heal all that suffer. This is the uncanny mark of the wounded healer.
Joan Halifax, *Shaman: The Wounded Healer*

We do not become healers. We came as healers. We are!
Some of us are still catching up to what we are.
Clarissa Pinkola Estés

I am, you are, a cell in a bigger living organism. We have been taught to forget this. But our bodies are remembering.

We are not the only ones who are suffering. We are not the only ones who are sick.

But we are the ones with the power to make a change.

The time has come to take back our power from this sickness.

It is time to purge the toxic masculine from our bodies and beings and planet. And to choose life.

Women are the life-bringers. And now we are bringing new life once again to the planet – a sustainable, healthier way of human life, one body at a time. One community at a time.

It is my belief that we are in fact medicine women for our culture – finding and bringing healing not only to ourselves but to those all around us.

We didn't consciously choose this role, but through it we are being transformed.

This era, it seems, is one of the vast initiation of the wounded healer, the medicine woman. People in their billions are looking for the leadership, the vision, the skills, tools and hope to know how to transform their suffering.

It is no coincidence that at the height of political uncertainty and environmental degradation we are being initiated in our millions to embody healing and transformation.

To be a wounded healer, in the philosophy of patriarchy, is to be weak, vulnerable, damaged, subjective, untrustworthy, faulty. To be a wounded healer in the Feminine is to have been touched by sacred suffering, to have been humbled, broken open, to have a deeper compassion and embodied empathy. The wounded healer is she who has learned how to transmute or transcend pain. She who is able to connect not only with her own pain, but is able to feel on behalf of her community. She who is connected to her own soul. She who is able to transform some of the suffering of a sick culture through her own body. She is one who is committed to dreaming on behalf of the Earth.

A medicine woman is not she who has never suffered or has never been broken. A medicine woman is she who does not uphold the denial of the world, but is a conduit for the mystery of beyond. She who is able to navigate in the dark. She who finds expression for what has lain silent, unspoken, unseen. She who listens and watches when others rush in. She who values healing – for herself, her children – above silence. Who values her health and wellbeing above invisibility and keeping others happy. Above worrying what others think. Above being an inconvenience. Above trying to fit in and be normal and not make a fuss. Above upholding the System.

A medicine woman is initiated into her own place in the cycle of life and is shown her own limitations and mortality clearly. She is humbled by her body and learns to transcend pain and suffering because of the physical and energetic limitations placed upon her. She does not become a victim to her illness, nor does she ignore or deny its impact on her body and her life. She learns the power of her mind and her body through her trials with them.

Those of us who develop the skills of knowing how to cope with massive inner change, with sickness and dissolution, we who learn to cope when things fall apart for ourselves and our families, build the skills and resources of resilience that will be so desperately needed in the coming years as the System collapses.

The next generation of medicine women is being initiated now.

Our time has come.

PREGNANT WITH A NEW WORLD

We did not know
When we first felt the pull of nausea, the ache in our bones,
That we were early-days pregnant with a new world.
But we were.
We are.
We are bringing forth newness from our bodies.
Medicine Woman
is our midwife, our doula,
She sits in the dark with us and waits.
Reminding us of the wisdom of the dark,
The power of the liminal,
Our own power to both transcend and surrender.
She reminds us of what we know in our bones.
She places her hand on our lower back to centre us.
And then she is gone again.
A scream in the dark,
A hand reaching out to us…
And we step into her place.
We are the medicine women.

MEDICINE QUESTIONS

Envisioning Health

Having read this book, can you create a visual representation of your big picture vision of your health? Not someone else's vision but your very own. Try not to make it too fluffy and aspirational, nor the generic capitalist vision of what health and wellbeing looks like at spas or ten-thousand-dollar yoga retreats or skinny muscular bodies. What does it really look and feel like to you? This might be harder than it first seems to move beyond what we have been sold as health, to what we actually long for.

Can you write it, draw it, collage it?

Now take a look at this image. What is standing between you and wellness? What is between your vision of yourself as healthy and vibrant and where you are now? How can you make your vision into a reality? What habits do you keep falling into and why? What are the stories you are telling yourself about why you can't do it now? Is it because you are tired, in pain, short of money, exhausted, overwhelmed? Is it because it feels foreign, stressful, tiring or just unfamiliar? How can you make it more comforting, desirable, easier, nourishing and accessible? How can you bring this vision to life?

Commit to trying one of the health-making behaviours you have listed within the next fortnight. Tell a friend or therapist so that you are accountable. How does it make you feel – during and after? How can you break more long-term goals down into individual actions? How do you want to track and celebrate your progress?

Your New Normal

What does your new normal look like?

What ways of interacting with the physical environment are not working for you?

How well does your spirituality, sexuality and creative practice answer the needs of your unique soul?

Where or how can you find and stay connected to safe people?

What is your marker of success? What are you aiming at, how will you know when you have got there? When or how will you decide to adapt the destination?

How can you come out about your experience and fully inhabit your lived reality more publicly?

How can you adapt your life to your needs?

Illness and Transformation

If you could wave a magic wand, what would you change?

What have you had to let go of?

What have you gained?

What skills or qualities has being sick developed in you?

How have you shared these with others?

How has fear featured in your illness?

What is your overriding expectation of yourself... and how has sickness impacted on this?

Look at your lineage – how much has sickness had a major part in the lives of your ancestors? How has it shaped their bodies, lives, relationships? What have you inherited from them – genetically, and in terms of beliefs? How do you feel about this?

What has being sick made you prioritise?

How do you treat your energy now?

What have you learned about yourself from being sick?

What have you learned about those close to you since being sick?

What have you learned about our culture since being sick?

Go through each area of your life: personal relationships, eating, exercise, leisure, hygiene, work, transport – how do they need to be in order to support you as you are now? What will you have to let go of from your old life to get there? How can you mourn that?

Bucket List

List thirty things that you love, that you've always wanted to do, that you keep telling yourself you'll do next year/when you are well/when the kids are grown up/when you have enough money/when you've lost the weight/when you're retired. Make sure they're things that you're passionate about now, not other people's dreams, and not the dreams of a former self of days gone by. They might be big or small.

Once you've written out the list (perhaps creatively with doodles and bright coloured pens) take a look over them. Which could you do now... but in an adapted way? So, if your mobility/finances/anxiety won't allow a real trip to a theme park any time soon, you might take a virtual ride on a roller-coaster using a phone and VR goggles, or via a first person POV film on You Tube. You may not be able to make it to the beach, but you could order some shells online and add them to your altar space, or watch a movie set at the sea.

And with those that are within your reach – set one as a goal, tell your closest folks and conspire together to make it possible.

THE HEALING REVOLUTION

*I must fight with all my strength so that the little positive things
that my health allows me to do might be pointed toward helping the
revolution: the only real reason for living.*
Frida Kahlo

*Once we are all ill and confined to the bed, [...] bearing witness to
each other's tales of trauma, prioritizing the care and love of our sick,
pained, expensive, sensitive, fantastic bodies, and there is no one left to
go to work, perhaps then, finally, capitalism will screech to its much-
needed, long-overdue, and motherfucking glorious halt.*
Johanna Hedva, "Sick Woman Theory"

I always had the sense that when The Revolution came, I would know
about it. We are used to Revolution being bloody: the man in the
street rising up and violently overthrowing his ideological adversaries.
What is happening now is far more subtle, so as to go almost unseen.
It is not the man on the street, but the woman in the bed, who is
throwing up, bleeding, falling and calling time on our culture. Sick
women are quietly making the sick System sit up and listen.

The Revolution is fomenting in Facebook groups as women mobilise resources, coach each other by Skype and Messenger, choose essential oils over antibiotics, psychological assessment over punishing their
children. Women who go armed with information seeking referrals
and demanding second opinions, who are taking chemo and crowd-
funding for complementary cancer treatment, who are demanding to
be heard, demanding the care they deserve, seeking out the support
they need for themselves and their children.

We imagined The Revolution would come one fine day, that some-one else would organise it, and we'd show up if it fitted into our over-packed schedules, if our health was good, the transport laid on, if our anxieties were low and the sun was shining. And we'd pack up our cleverly-worded placards and march.

Instead we find we are in the midst of the chaos, feeling sick and anxious, limbs aching, knowing that change needs to happen and now, for us all. But we find that there's no clear vision, no clear leader, no guaranteed alternatives, no shining path to utopia. All we're being told is that there's not enough money. Not enough staff. Not enough to go around. The System is broken. We have to join a waiting list. So we wait, and wait. And wait. And get sicker and sicker.

Or we pay if we can, borrowing money from friends, family, lenders, remortgaging our home, selling our car. Or we pull the money from our savings, or the pension pot, we cut the health insurance that we need but can't afford.

And we wait. And make do. We tolerate our pain a little longer. And then we wait some more.

For someone to save us.

And then one day we notice that Medicine Woman has thoughtfully emptied out our schedules so that the only thing on our agenda is to fight for our health, individually, collectively. She has thrown a stick in the wheels of industry so that we show up.

We thought The Revolution would come some day when we were ready.

This is The Revolution, sisters.
Right here and now.
It's started from the inside.
The life on the line is yours.
This bed, this sofa, this hospital ward, this doctor's waiting room is your healing field.
The time for fighting in the old way is done.
It is time for a revolution in healing.
We are the resistance,
We occupy our bodies, our feelings, our minds,

And dedicate ourselves to reclaiming our mother tongue,
The language of our bodies and our feelings.
We occupy ourselves.
Reclaiming the System for our systems,
Remembering our power.
Declaring the wild body to be wise, the wild mind sovereign territory.
We are pioneers,
Mapping the terrain as we move through it,
No longer following the route labelled normal and bending our contours to fit it.
In a world that would name us,
We choose to name ourselves.
In a world that would silence our suffering, ignore our difference,
We dare to wear our labels with pride.
In a world that would call us victims, patients,
We declare at last
That we are the medicine women
And it is time to heal.

EPILOGUE

People want a triumphant narrative. They want to know that you have solved the problem of your body. But my body is not a problem and it's certainly not something I have solved yet.[129]

Roxane Gay

This book has been a lesson in bravery. In my own strength and vulnerability. In showing up to my biggest fears, both in my bodymind and in the world. It has broken and humbled me on a daily basis.

What I have learned in the process is that bravery is a daily practice. At its heart it is the practice of reaching for love in the face of unrelenting fear. Courage looks different on different days – some days it is staying alive minute by minute, other days it is making an appointment, or showing up for it. Some days it is taking a pill, other days it is choosing not to.

And some days it is hitting publish on a book.

I cursed this sickness for taking from me the life I loved: unable to be in the world, to move, to read, to write, to mother, to work. But in truth it reconnected me with all these things on a deeper level. The sickness did not take me from my work, it led me further into it.

I have learned a lot over the course of these past two and a half years. A very different woman is writing these words to the one who started it.

I began this book aware of some of the puzzle pieces I may be dealing with. But not knowing how to slot them together. No doctor had ever managed to either. I felt like I couldn't turn up to this book without a definite diagnosis. Later I felt I couldn't finish it without a cure.

In the end it took several years of my own research and finding specialists in the field to be able to tell me what was wrong. To give me the gold-plated diagnosis of most of the pieces. Others are still hypotheses. There are no cures within Western medicine for many of my ailments, so whilst I am healing and much more functional, I am not cured.

I hold out hope for the future. The day I finished writing the final draft I stumbled upon a grand unifying theory, proposed by a female medical doctor and chronic health sufferer, that is currently being studied by geneticists. It explores the connections between the symptoms that I and so many women featured in this book and our families, share: a genetic mutation which makes us especially susceptible to stress. A mutation that explains why so many women have clusters of co-morbid conditions, why joint hypermobility, anxiety, chronic fatigue, autism, irritable bowel and migraine appear together. In short, she posits a genetic hypothesis for why some of us are so sick. It is early days, but it makes sense to me. And so I share her website here and will keep an eye on how it develops: www.rccxandillness.com

Writing and living the *Medicine Woman* journey has been the hardest thing I have ever done. I am under no illusions that it is perfect. But it is here. And I am here. Neither of those things were in any way guaranteed as the process unfurled.

And you, my love, are here too. So if you leave these pages with a sense of not being alone in your suffering, if it has helped to alleviate some of your fear, if it has helped shed light on the inner process going on as you navigate sickness, and the outer journey of navigating the broken System, if it has helped in some way show you more of the puzzle pieces, or even put a few together, then I am happy I was brave.

Here's to our healing,

Lucy H. Pearce,

Cork, Ireland, August 2018

APPENDICES

A NOTE ON TERMS

Words… they can be tricky things. The right one can unlock a door in the mind, connect the dots, switch on a light. The wrong one can close the door to shared understanding, and make a reader slam a book shut. There are some terms that I use frequently that may be unfamiliar or challenging to you, I want to explain my reasoning for them briefly here. Think of these concepts and words as the main characters of the book, and this is where you get to meet them.

Use of Capitalisation

When terms such as Medicine Woman, the System and the Feminine are capitalised they refer to the archetypal understanding of a concept (following the style of *Burning Woman*). When I refer to a human individual who is embodying an archetype, the term is not capitalised, so a masseuse or doctor may be referred to as a medicine woman.

Archetype: To me, Medicine Woman is an archetype, a universal energetic blueprint, which though it may differ subtly from culture to culture, is common to all humans, just like the idea of a Mother, Teacher or Queen would be. The focus of my work is on reclaiming lost archetypes of the Feminine – energies which have been forgotten, side-lined, ignored or buried during patriarchal times, but which hold great power for us in these transition times as we imagine new ways forward. Different people approach archetypes in different ways. For some it may help to imagine an archetype as real, a living, breathing otherworldly inhabitant, a spirit or aspect of the Goddess. For others, it is an energy force that can be tapped into and released into our world when we embody its qualities. For others it is merely a metaphor, an idea which can inspire us.

Bodymind: This term is used throughout this book and may be new to you. Popularised by Ken Dychtwald in his book, *Bodymind*, it seeks to linguistically close the artificial schism between body and mind within Western culture and instead approach the human being holistically. This is not just a happy hippie way of looking at things, but at the forefront of what science is discovering: "The interaction of Psyche and Soma are well known and this interaction happens through a complex network of feedback, medication, and modulation among the central and autonomic nervous systems, the endocrine system, the immune system, and the stress system. These systems, which were previously considered pristinely independent, in fact, interact at myriad levels. Psychoneuroimmunology (PNI) is an emerging discipline that focuses on various interactions among these body systems and provides the underpinnings of a scientific explanation for what is commonly referred to as the mind-body connection."[130] *Psyche and soma: New insights into the connection*, Rahul Kumar and Vikram K. Yeragani

Healing Ally: I use this term to cover any being who is working with you in a healing capacity – whatever field they work in, professional or not, human or not. A healing ally is someone who is positively partnering you on your healing journey.

Medicine Woman: Many cultures have their own understanding of Medicine Woman, the native healer outside of the Western medical tradition, and their own earthly lineages of her apprentices: medicine people with closely guarded rituals, skills in herbs, abilities to speak with spirits and lay on hands. They may be known as the shaman, the wise woman, the witch, the healer, the priestess, the midwife, the wyrd woman.

The person who works with the understanding of Medicine Woman, whatever their heritage or tradition is, in my eyes, a medicine woman, or man.

My understanding of Medicine Woman – both the human healer and the archetypal understanding – is careful not to appropriate any other culture's practices, nor recreate some naïvely imagined lost past, but is rather breathing deeper understanding into a commonly used term that many women from many cultures feel an innate resonance with. We can learn humbly from other cultures those things that our own has forgotten, yes, but more importantly it is about re-establishing our own organic, native connection with our innate healing ability, our own landscapes, and actively questioning and rebalancing the masculine dominance of Western medicine in our own bodyminds and communities. We do not seek to take what is not ours. We seek to heal, to whole, to find what was lost, forgotten, abandoned, denied. We seek to uncover what was hidden. To remember. Deeply. Who we are and why we are here.

Paradigm: The word paradigm comes from the Greek for 'pattern', it is a map or model of reality. A 'paradigm shift', a term coined by philosopher of science Thomas Kuhn in the 1970s, is a fundamental shift in our understanding of the way things are, our approach or underlying assumptions.

Psyche/Soul: The term 'soul' is often only used in religious or spiritual contexts. The way that it is used in this book is as an acknowledgement of ourselves beyond the physical body. It is an attempt to express in a single word the innate *beingness* of each of us that cannot be touched or photographed but which is the true expression and experience of ourselves.

The etymology of psyche is "animating spirit," from the Latin *psyche* and from Greek *psykhe,* "the soul, mind, spirit; breath; life, one's life, the invisible animating principle or entity which occupies and directs the physical body."[131]

Psychic: I use this term to refer to things of the psyche, not mind-reading skills.

The Feminine: The feminine/Feminine, can be a term that many find challenging. I get it. Please refer to my words from *Burning Woman* just in case it is a term you struggle with too:

Whatever gender we were assigned at birth, we all have both 'masculine' and 'feminine' energies and drives within us. And we're all born into a patriarchal culture which sees and shapes us differently into stunted, restricted versions of the full people we could be.

'The feminine' as it is currently used in our culture is usually short-hand for: beautiful, gentle, slim, restrained, non-confrontational, carefully cultivated, domesticated, emotional, girlish and weak. It is often a term of disparagement... because the feminine has been black-listed. Most qualities deemed not masculine, or in any way pertaining to women, have been slighted, shamed or silenced.

Both genders in our culture have learned to suppress signs of the feminine in order to survive and be accepted, which has led to a hyper-masculinised culture of men... and women. As women in Western culture we have been taught to value more masculine traits and denigrate, disregard or trivialise more typically feminine ways of being.

So let's differentiate now by using a capital F. The Feminine is your deepest life-force which is expressed through your female body. It is that which feels most true to you as a woman: uncultivated and raw.

Defining the Feminine is immediately problematic – it sets up a dichotomy with the Masculine. And in this world, we have a habit of making dichotomies into good and bad.

The reality we are currently inhabiting is the shadowlands where immature masculine and feminine are waiting transformation into a creative partnership of their fully mature selves.

The masculinity we see running rampant in the patriarchal system is not the developed Masculine, but the defensive toxic masculine, the immature, ego-based masculine trying to defend a man-made hierarchical order against chaos, nature and the Feminine.

The System and The Patriarchy: We inhabit a System that has been constructed, ruled over and policed for millennia by men, prioritising the needs, perspectives, bodies and minds of men. The System (often referred to as patriarchy in feminist thought) has forcibly separated humanity down gendered and sexed divides. It has violently enforced the primacy of what it recognises as the male and the masculine whilst devaluing, destroying and suppressing that which it defines as female and feminine. We must of course be clear that the term 'patriarchy' does not mean that men as individuals are bad or wrong or inherently guilty. After all men suffer at the hands of patriarchy too. And many women claim to not even experience it at all.

Whether we consciously acknowledge it or not, patriarchy is the paradigm in which our bodies have grown, our lives have been shaped, our health managed and our minds bound for tens of generations. It has controlled, ordered and interpreted our lives across religious, political and cultural fields in consciously gendered ways that have systemically and historically discriminated against women. Our current System is informed by three main strands of patriarchy: the patriarchy of the mind – law, the patriarchy of the body – medical science, and the patriarchy of the soul – the Church.

Western Medicine: I have thought long and hard about how to refer to the dominant scientific medical paradigm in this book, not wanting to cement the artificial divide between 'East' and 'West', aware that most countries around the world now prioritise 'Western' medical approaches. And also aware that many pioneering technologies are coming from 'Eastern' countries like India, China, Korea and Japan. I have decided upon Western medicine, to acknowledge its roots in both ancient Roman and Greek philosophy as well as the European scientific tradition.

CONTEXTUALISING THE SYSTEM

Health and healing are such emotive topics, with so many diverse perspectives, informed by our personal experiences, educations and values. The first part of the book explores The System, which will look different to you depending on where you live and who you are. It is also subject to change, depending on who is holding power within the political system at any time. Nevertheless, within patriarchal capitalist countries, the System is similar enough that local discrepancies are really only the flavour – patriarchy is the ice cream we're all eating.

The System I live in is the Irish System. I was born here, but spent my childhood in the UK, coming back to settle here with my first baby in my womb, and a very English accent. As a consequence I have a lived experience of the good and bad parts of the UK National Health Service – a socialised form of health care, free at the point of access, but hugely underinvested in and with lengthy waiting lists. I have family and many friends in America, so have observed from the outside the ups and downs of this System, with the most advanced medical treatment in the world, but which comes at a truly terrifying financial cost, out of reach of so many, and with a massive reliance on pharmaceutical medication.

In Ireland our System is a combination between a public system, similar to, but not nearly as extensive as the NHS, which you can receive free of charge if your income is low enough and an extensive private health system which runs in parallel where health insurance is the norm and much more affordable than in the US. Most families, except the very poorest, would access aspects of private healthcare regularly because many things are not available publicly, and waiting lists on public services can run to years. The waiting list for diagnosis for autism is eighteen to twenty-four months, for a therapist I waited fourteen months. At the time of writing the region next to us announced that from the following month they would have no child psychiatrists employed on the public system, as their three had all left.

As a small country of just over 4 million people, Ireland has a complete lack of consultants and specialist doctors in many areas of medicine, and patients regularly must visit specialists in the UK, Europe or US. Families often have to leave the country to avail of medications which are not legal here such as medical marijuana or abortion pills.

Another factor of the Irish healthcare system is the involvement of the Catholic Church. When I was born in 1980 it was nuns who delivered me in the city maternity hospital (my family are not Catholic). Many hospitals were established on Church-owned lands, and have Church representatives on the board of management that still have a direct say in what may or may not happen in the hospital. Homebirth was made technically illegal here when I was pregnant with my second child, by removing insurance from homebirth midwives. Myself and several other pregnant mothers had to conduct a nationwide campaign in the national media, parliament and with the heads of the Health Service Executive in order to get it reinstated.

During the writing of this book abortion was legalised in Ireland. Previous to this women faced the issue of mandatory pregnancy testing before many medications were administered, including those for MS or bipolar. A positive test would mean the discontinuation of the medication, as the life of the foetus held the same legal rights as that of the mother. Medical professionals could not act to save the life of a pregnant woman if their actions would potentially kill her unborn child. Contraception was only legalised here in 1980 to prescription holders and only made freely available in 1995. Thousands of women during the past century were forced to go to mother and baby homes, run by the Catholic Church, their babies forcibly adopted, the mothers shamed and used as slave labour under humiliating conditions.

As I finished editing this book, another scandal in women's health broke, where it was discovered that the national cervical cancer screening program had discovered an issue with many false negative results over the course of several years, and had deliberately withheld this information from women and their families. Women who were now dying from the disease. Women's healthcare here is better than it has ever been... but as you can see, this is not hard. To be a woman here is still to be navigating the System differently.

I am aware that some readers will identify with my frustrations at the public health system, others will have no experience of socialised health care. Some will understand the cost of private healthcare or the impact of religious bodies on it, others will not.

I chose not include this information in the main body of the book, as my readership is international, and these cases are particular to Ireland, but feel it is important to share it here so that you know the context within which I write.

REFERENCES

1   www.cwhn.ca/en/resources/primers/chronicdisease

2   www.aarda.org/autoimmune-information/autoimmune-disease-in-women

3   www.aarda.org/knowledge-base/women-susceptible-autoimmune-disease-men

4   www.diapedia.org/type-1-diabetes-mellitus/2104085168/
    epidemiology-of-type-1-diabetes

5   www.aarda.org/knowledge-base/
    specific-autoimmune-diseases-affect-women-men

6   www.sharecare.com/health/fibromyalgia/
    percentage-population-affected-by-fibromyalgia

7   www.aarda.org/knowledge-base/
    specific-autoimmune-diseases-affect-women-men

8   www.ncbi.nlm.nih.gov/pubmed/8578167

9   www.newyorker.com/magazine/2013/08/26/whats-wrong-with-me

10 www.aarda.org/who-we-help/patients/women-and-autoimmunity

11 www.diapedia.org/type-1-diabetes-mellitus/2104085168/
    epidemiology-of-type-1-diabetes

12 www.aarda.org/who-we-help/patients/women-and-autoimmunity

13 www.newyorker.com/magazine/2013/08/26/whats-wrong-with-me

14 Maya Dusenbery. *Doing Harm: The Truth About How Bad Medicine and Lazy
    Science Leave Women Dismissed, Misdiagnosed, and Sick.*

15 www.aarda.org/who-we-help/patients/women-and-autoimmunity

16 broadly.vice.com/en_us/article/gy899x/
    maya-dusenbery-how-doctors-gaslight-women-doubting-their-own-pain

17 www.theguardian.com/environment/2018/jul/18/
    asthma-deaths-rise-25-amid-growing-air-pollution-crisis

18 www.theguardian.com/environment/2016/aug/29/declare-anthropocene-
    epoch-experts-urge-geological-congress-human-impact-earth

19 www.theguardian.com/environment/2018/jul/23/
    rising-temperatures-linked-to-increased-suicide-rates

20   www.theguardian.com/environment/2016/jun/13/
air-pollution-linked-to-increased-mental-illness-in-children

21   Centers for Disease Control and Prevention, reported in
www.theguardian.com/society/commentisfree/2018/jul/19/
drugs-alone-wont-fix-our-epidemic-of-depression

22   www.diapedia.org/type-1-diabetes-mellitus/2104085168/
epidemiology-of-type-1-diabetes

23   See Anthony William, *Medical Medium*

24   www.theguardian.com/business/2016/may/16/
uk-poverty-rates-office-for-national-statistics

25   www.theguardian.com/us-news/2017/jun/28/
womens-healthcare-republican-senate-bill

26   www.who.int/mental_health/prevention/genderwomen/en/

27   www.theguardian.com/inequality/2018/feb/17/
dirty-secret-why-housework-gender-gap

28   www.aauw.org/research/the-simple-truth-about-the-gender-pay-gap/

29   onbeing.org/blog/the-disease-of-being-busy

30   Heath, Sarah. p156 in *The Nine Degrees of Autism*, Philip Wylie et al.

31   Elizabeth Sewell, referenced in Wilentz, *Healing Narratives: Women Writers Curing Cultural Dis-ease.*

32   www.newyorker.com/magazine/2013/08/26/whats-wrong-with-me

33   www.theguardian.com/society/2018/jun/29/
women-often-feel-patronised-by-doctors-health-minister-says

34   www.theguardian.com/society/2018/jul/20/
cervical-cancer-testing-drive-will-aim-to-tackle-huge-surge-in-no-shows

35   breastcancernow.org/news-and-blogs/news/breast-cancer-now-responds-to-
new-figures-showing-uptake-of-nhs-breast-screening-falls-to-decade-low

36   www.england.nhs.uk/atlas_case_study/improving-vaccination-uptake-by-
changing-the-way-pregnant-women-were-offered-and-accessed-services/

37   www.the-pool.com/health/health/2018/26/
Anna-Hart-on-getting-a-dyspraxia-diagnosis-as-adult-woman

38   kindredmedia.org/2018/06/ending-patriarchy/

39   Foucault. *Madness and Civilization.*

40   18th century doctor, Van Helmut, quoted in Foucault, *Madness and Civilization.*

41   en.wikipedia.org/wiki/List_of_medical_roots,_suffixes_and_prefixes

42   www.etymonline.com/word/psyche

43   en.wikipedia.org/wiki/Asclepius

44 The modern version of the Hippocratic Oath was written in 1964 by Louis Lasagna, Dean of the School of Medicine at Tufts University. Sourced from www.medicinenet.com/script/main/art.asp?articlekey=20909

45 The classical version of the Hippocratic Oath is from the translation from the Greek by Ludwig Edelstein. From *The Hippocratic Oath: Text, Translation, and Interpretation*, by Ludwig Edelstein.

46 Agnew, John "Deus Vult: The Geopolitics of Catholic Church". Geopolitics. 15 (1): 39–61. doi:10.1080/14650040903420388.

47 Catholic News Agency. 10 February 2010.

48 Alexander Armstrong, Italy's Invisible Cities, BBC.

49 Foucault. *Madness and Civilization*.

50 Foucault. *Madness and Civilization*.

51 "Man a Machine" (1747), Julien Offray De La Mettrie.

52 Gilbert Ryle's description of René Descartes' mind-body dualism, a term popularised by Arthur Koestler in his 1967 work of philosophical psychology, *The Ghost in the Machine*.

53 www.slate.com/articles/health_and_science/medical_examiner/2013/04/ diagnostic_and_statistical_manual_fifth_edition_why_will_half_the_u_s_ population.html

54 Thanks to Patrick Treacy for the insight on this.

55 See Ferguson, Marilyn. *The Aquarian Conspiracy*.

56 Horwitz, Allan and Jerome Wakefield, *The Loss of Sadness: How Psychiatry Transformed Normal Sorrow into Depressive Disorder.*

57 www.theguardian.com/society/2018/mar/10/ panic-chronic-anxiety-burnout-doctors-breaking-point

58 Sontag, Susan. *Illness as Metaphor.*

59 Ward BW, Schiller JS, Goodman RA. Multiple chronic conditions among US adults: a 2012 update: dx.doi.org/10.5888/pcd11.130389

60 www.cdc.gov/chronicdisease

61 digital.nhs.uk/article/3199/More-than-1-billion-prescription-items-dispensed-in-a-year---or-1900-a-minute

62 2017 figure based on United Nations estimate.

63 www.cdc.gov/nchs/fastats/drug-use-therapeutic.htm

64 www.usnews.com/news/best-states/vermont/articles/2018-02-08/ vermont-committee-supports-canadian-prescription-drug-plan

65 www.theguardian.com/society/2018/jun/03/ precision-medicine-breast-cancer-remove-need-chemotherapy

66 www.ncbi.nlm.nih.gov/books/NBK223657

67 www.theguardian.com/society/commentisfree/2018/jul/19/
drugs-alone-wont-fix-our-epidemic-of-depression

68 www.bostonglobe.com/opinion/2014/01/05/every-cell-has-sex/
lgnbRyR1FvVqA9ccbKM5iI/story.html and https://www.theguardian.com/
lifeandstyle/2015/apr/30/fda-clinical-trials-gender-gap-epa-nih-institute-of-
medicine-cardiovascular-disease

69 www.ted.com/talks/alyson_mcgregor_why_medicine_
often_has_dangerous_side_effects_for_women/
transcript

70 See Ferguson, Marilyn. *The Aquarian Conspiracy.*

71 www.reuters.com/article/us-health-physicians-pay-gaps/pay-gaps-persist-for-
female-and-african-american-physicians-in-us-idUSKBN1HI1E0

72 www.theguardian.com/science/2016/feb/15/
jo-marchant-mind-body-health-medicine-science

73 www.samhsa.gov

74 www.drugabuse.gov/drugs-abuse/opioids/opioid-crisis

75 www.theguardian.com/us-news/2017/oct/19/
big-pharma-money-lobbying-us-opioid-crisis

76 www.washingtonpost.com/graphics/2017/investigations/
dea-drug-industry-congress/?utm_term=.3ecbea861420

77 edition.cnn.com/2017/09/18/health/opioid-crisis-fast-facts/index.html

78 www.theguardian.com/us-news/2018/may/26/
traces-of-opioids-found-in-mussels-in-seattle-bay

79 See *Bridges of the Bodymind.*

80 See tinyurl.com/reasonsforwomen for the dozens of different reasons given for
incarcerating women in mental asylums in the mid nineteenth century.

81 broadly.vice.com/en_us/article/gy899x/
maya-dusenbery-how-doctors-gaslight-women-doubting-their-own-pain

82 www.theatlantic.com/health/archive/2015/10/
emergency-room-wait-times-sexism/410515/

83 Foucault. *Madness and Civilization.*

84 Hoffman, Diane E. "The Girl Who Cried Pain: A Bias Against Women in the
Treatment of Pain."

85 Ibid.

86 www.nytimes.com/2018/05/03/well/live/when-doctors-downplay-womens-
health-concerns.html

87 Bethany Webster. Womb of Light.com

88 Stephen Ilardi – Kessler et al 2005.

89 www.theguardian.com/science/2018/feb/21/
the-drugs-do-work-antidepressants-are-effective-study-shows

90   www.theguardian.com/society/2017/apr/14/
      one-in-four-young-women-in-uk-report-mental-health-issues-study-shows

91   www.theguardian.com/society/2018/aug/10/
      four-million-people-in-england-are-long-term-users-of-antidepressants

92   en.wikipedia.org/wiki/Women_in_medicine

93   www.theguardian.com/world/2018/aug/02/
      tokyo-medical-school-changed-test-scores-to-keep-women-out

94   www.theguardian.com/world/2018/aug/08/
      tokyo-medical-school-admits-changing-results-to-exclude-women

95   www.thejournal.ie/female-doctors-ireland-1046065-Aug2013/

96   www.nhs.uk/NHSEngland/thenhs/about/Pages/overview.aspx

97   www.nhsemployers.org/~/media/Employers/Publications/Gender%20in%20
      the%20NHS

98   Ibid.

99   Ibid.

100   www.theguardian.com/healthcare-network/2017/mar/01/
      why-so-few-male-nurses

101   www.theguardian.com/society/2018/jun/29/
      women-often-feel-patronised-by-doctors-health-minister-says

102   www.reuters.com/article/us-health-physicians-pay-gaps/pay-gaps-persist-for-
      female-and-african-american-physicians-in-us-idUSKBN1HI1E0

103   minoritynurse.com/nursing-statistics/

104   www.psychologytoday.com/us/blog/
      here-there-and-everywhere/201701/11-warning-signs-gaslighting

105   uk.businessinsider.com/
      what-is-karoshi-japanese-word-for-death-by overwork-2017-10

106   Sky News 1/7/2018.

107   Brewer, Joe. "The Pain You Feel is Capitalism Dying" – Medium.com

108   "Differences between Male and Female Consumers of Complementary and
      Alternative Medicine in a National US Population: A Secondary Analysis of
      2012 NIHS Data" www.hindawi.com/journals/ecam/2015/413173/

109   Ibid.

110   en.wikipedia.org/wiki/Paradigm_shift

111   See Mehl-Madrona, Lewis. *Narrative Medicine: The Use of History and Story in
      the Healing Process.*

112   tealswan.com/resources/articles/what-is-healing-r285/

113   brenebrown.com/blog/2018/05/24/the-midlife-unraveling/

114   van der Kolk, Bessel. *The Body Keeps the Score.*

115   brenebrown.com/blog/2018/05/24/the-midlife-unraveling/

116 Miserandino, Christine. "The Spoon Theory", www.butyoudontlooksick.com/articles/written-by-christine/the-spoon-theory

117 From eco-philosopher Joanna Macy.

118 www.explorejournal.com/article/S1550-8307(08)00285-1/fulltext

119 www.nytimes.com/2018/01/27/opinion/sunday/surgery-germany-vicodin.html

120 myheartsisters.org/2014/06/08/convalescence/

121 Woodman, Marion. *Leaving My Father's House.*

122 See Greer, Carl. *Change Your Story, Change Your Life: using shamanic and Jungian tools to achieve personal transformation* and Mehl-Madrona, *Lewis. Narrative Medicine: The Use of History and Story in the Healing Process.*

123 www.stuff.co.nz/national/102115864/in-narrative-therapy-mori-creation-stories-are-being-used-to-heal

124 www.welcometocountry.org/traditional-aboriginal-healers-australia-hospitals

125 For more on this approach see Hay, Louise L. *You Can Heal Your Life.*

126 See *Bridges of the Bodymind.*

127 marthabeck.com/2010/10/creativity-tips-from-martha/

128 badwitch.es/women-society-calls-damaged-powerful

129 Roxane Gay interviewed by Trevor Noah quoted in heatherplett.com/2017/06/body-without-triumphant-narrative

130 www.ncbi.nlm.nih.gov/pmc/articles/PMC3146208/

131 www.etymonline.com/word/psyche

RESOURCES

BOOKS

Personal, Creative and Literary Memoir of Illness and Healing

Duff, Kat. *The Alchemy of Illness.*

Ensler, Eve. *In the Body of the World: A Memoir of Cancer and Connection.*

Forster, Margaret. *Lady's Maid.*

Gay, Roxane. *Hunger: A Memoir of (My) Body.*

Gilman, Charlotte Perkins. *The Yellow Wallpaper.*

Gill, Nikita, *Wild Embers.*

Hustvedt, Siri. *The Shaking Woman.*

Jung, C.G. *The Red Book.*

Kahlo, Frida. *The Diary of Frida Kahlo.*

Lorde, Audre. *A Burst of Light and other essays.*

Morrow Lindbergh, Anne. *Gift from the Sea.*

Pearce, Lucy H. *Moods of Motherhood: The Inner Journey of Mothering.*

Picoult, Jodi. *Second Glance.*

Plath, Sylvia. *Ariel.*

Plath, Sylvia. *The Bell Jar.*

Rukeyser, Muriel. "Double Ode", in *The Collected Poems of Muriel Rukeyser.*

Sontag, Susan. *Illness as Metaphor.*

Strayed, Cheryl. *Wild.*

Woolf, Virginia. *On Being Ill.*

Women's Health

Boston Women's Health Collective. *Our Bodies, Ourselves.*

Dusenbery, Maya. *Doing Harm: The Truth About How Bad Medicine and Lazy Science Leave Women Dismissed, Misdiagnosed, and Sick.*

Gottfried, Dr. Sara. *The Hormone Cure: Reclaim Balance, Sleep, Sex Drive and Vitality Naturally with the Gottfried Protocol.*

Kent, Tami Lynn. *Wild Feminine: Finding Power, Spirit and Joy in the Female Body.*

Northrup, Dr. Christiane. *Women's Bodies, Women's Wisdom: Creating Physical and Emotional Health and Healing.*

Pearce, Lucy H. *Full Circle Health: Integrated Health Charting for Women.*

Pearce, Lucy H. *Moon Time: Harness the Ever-Changing Energy of your Menstrual Cycle.*

Pope, Alexandra Pope and Sjanie Hugo Wurlitzer. *Wild Power: Discover the Magic of Your Menstrual Cycle and Awaken the Feminine Path to Power.*

Shore, Lesley. *Healing the Feminine: Reclaiming Woman's Voice.*

Shuttle, Penelope and Peter Redgrove. *Alchemy for Women: Personal Transformation Through Dreams and the Female Cycle.*

Weed, Susun S. *Healing Wise: The Wise Woman Herbal.*

Woodman, Marion. *Leaving My Father's House: A Journey to Conscious Femininity.*

Youmell, Paula and Jenny Morrill. *Weaving Healing Wisdom.*

Autoimmune Conditions

Edwards, Laurie. *In the Kingdom of the Sick: A Social History of Chronic Illness in America.*

Jackson Nakazawa, Donna. *The Autoimmune Epidemic.*

Maté, Gabor. *When the Body Says No: Exploring the Stress-Disease Connection.*

Stoff, Jesse and Charles R. Pellegrino. *Chronic Fatigue Syndrome – The Hidden Epidemic.*

Oxytocin, Adrenaline and Trauma

Jackson Nakazawa, Donna. *Childhood Disrupted: How Your Biography Becomes Your Biology, and How You Can Heal.*

Levine, Peter. *In an Unspoken Voice: How the Body Releases Trauma and Restores Goodness.*

Levine, Peter. *Trauma and Memory: Brain and Body in a Search for the Living Past: A Practical Guide for Understanding and Working with Traumatic Memory.*

Miller, Alice. *The Body Never Lies: The Lingering Effects of Cruel Parenting.*

Miller, Alice. *The Drama of the Gifted Child: The Search for the True Self.*

Moberg Kerstin. *The Oxytocin Factor.*

Odent, Michel. *Childbirth in the Age of Plastic.*

van der Kolk, Bessel. *The Body Keeps the Score: Mind, Brain and Body in the Transformation of Trauma.*

Asperger's, Autism and Sensory Processing Issues in Women

Aron, Elaine M. *The Highly Sensitive Person: How to Thrive When the World Overwhelms You.*

Heller, Sharon. *Too Loud, Too Bright, Too Fast, Too Tight: What to Do If You Are Sensory Defensive in an Overstimulating World.*

Hendrickx, Sarah. *Women and Girls with Autism Spectrum Disorder: Understanding Life Experiences from Early Childhood to Old Age.*

Marshall, Tania A. *I Am Aspien Woman: The Unique Characteristics, Traits, and Gifts of Adult Females on the Autism Spectrum.*

Simone, Rudy. *Aspergirls: Empowering Females with Asperger Syndrome.*

Wylie, Philip et al. *The Nine Degrees of Autism: A Developmental Model for the Alignment and Reconciliation of Hidden Neurological Conditions.*

History of Medicine

Appignanesi, Lisa. *Mad, Bad and Sad: A History of Women and the Mind Doctors from 1800 to the Present.*

Barcan, Ruth. *Complementary and Alternative Medicine: Cultural Practice and the Boundaries of the Senses.*

Conrad, Peter. *The Medicalization of Society: On the Transformation of Human Conditions into Treatable Disorders.*

Ehrenreich, Barbara and Deirdre English. *Witches, Midwives and Nurses: A History of Women Healers.*

Farber, Seth. *The Spiritual Gift of Madness: The Failure of Psychiatry and the Rise of the Mad Pride Movement.*

Foucault, Michel. *Madness and Civilization: A History of Insanity in the Age of Reason.*

Foucault, Michel. *The Birth of The Clinic: An Archaeology of Medical Perception.*

Illich, Ivan. *Limits to Medicine: Medical Nemesis – The Expropriation of Health.*

Kuhn, Thomas. *The Structure of Scientific Revolutions.*

Leder, Drew. *The Absent Body.*

Penguin, *The Portable Enlightenment Reader.*

Showalter, Elaine. *Hystories: Hysterical Epidemics and Modern Culture.*

Showalter, Elaine. *The Female Malady: Women, Madness and English Culture 1830-1980.*

Literary and Cultural Theory

Daly, Mary. *Gyn/ecology: The Metaethics of Radical Feminism.*

Davies, William. *The Happiness Industry: How the Government and Big Business Sold Us Wellbeing.*

Doyal, Leslie. *What Makes Women Sick: Gender and the Political Economy of Health.*

Ehrenreich, Barbara. *Smile or Die: How Positive Thinking Fooled America and the World.*

Ferguson, Marilyn. *The Aquarian Conspiracy.*

Fromm, Erich. *The Sane Society.*

Johnson, Sharon D. (ed) *Seeing in the Dark: Wisdom Works by Black Women in Depth Psychology.*

Klein, Naomi. *The Shock Doctrine: The Rise of Disaster Capitalism.*

Lorde, Audre. *Sister Outsider.*

Moraga, Cherrie and Gloria Anzaldua (eds.) *This Bridge Called my Back, Fourth Edition: Writings by Radical Women of Color.*

Olorenshaw, Vanessa. *Liberating Motherhood: Birthing the Purplestockings Revolution.*

Pearce, Lucy H. *Burning Woman.*

Penelope, Julia. *Language and Metaphor.*

Sontag, Susan. *Illness as Metaphor.*

Wilentz, Gay. *Healing Narratives: Women Writers Curing Cultural Dis-ease.*

Woodman, Marion. *Conscious Femininity: Interviews with Marion Woodman.*

Wilkinson, Richard and Kate Pickett. *The Spirit Level: Why Greater Equality Makes Societies Stronger.*

Alternative Approaches to Health and Healing

Achterberg, Jeanne and G. Frank Lawlis. *Bridges of the Bodymind: Behavioural Approaches to Healthcare.*

Catto, Jamie. *Insanely Gifted: Turn Your Demons into Rocket Fuel.*

Dychtwald, Ken. *Bodymind.*

Estés, Dr. Clarissa Pinkola. *Women Who Run with the Wolves: Myths and Stories of the Wild Woman Archetype.*

Greer, Carl. *Change your Story, Change your Life: Using Shamanic and Jungian Tools to Achieve Personal Transformation.*

Hari, Johann. *Lost Connections: Uncovering the Real Causes of Depression – and the Unexpected Solutions.*

Hay, Louise L. *You Can Heal Your Life.*

Janov, Dr. Arthur. *The New Primal Scream: Primal Scream Therapy Twenty Years On.*

Judith, Anodea. *Eastern Body, Western Mind: Psychology and the Chakra System as a Path to the Self.*

Malachiodi, Cathy A. *The Art Therapy Sourcebook.*

Marchant, Jo. *Cure: A Journey into the Science of Mind over Body.*

McNiff, Shaun. *Art as Medicine.*

Mehl-Madrona, Lewis. *Narrative Medicine: The Use of History and Story in the Healing Process.*

Pearse, Innes, H. and Lucy H. Crocker. *The Peckham Experiment: A Study of the Living Structure of Society.*

Segal, Inna. *The Secret Language of your Body: The Essential Guide to Health and Wellness.*

Shapiro, Deb. *The Bodymind Workbook: Exploring How the Mind and Body Work Together.*

Tedlock, Barbara. *The Woman in the Shaman's Body: Reclaiming the Feminine in Religions and Medicine.*

William, Anthony. *Medical Medium: Secrets Behind Chronic and Mystery Illness and How to Finally Heal.*

Youmell, Paula. *Hands on Health: Take Your Vibrant, Whole Health Back into Your Healing Hands.*

Psyche – Mind and Soul

Bammel Wilding, Amy. *Wild & Wise: Sacred Feminine Meditations for Women's Circles and Personal Awakening.*

Bolen, Jean Shinoda. *Goddesses in Everywoman: A New Psychology of Women.*

Erickson, Victoria. *Rhythms & Roads.*

Grof, Stanislav. *Spiritual Emergency.*

Ingerman, Sandra. *Soul Retrieval: Mending the Fragmented Self.*

Jung, C.G. *Modern Man in Search of a Soul.*

Jung, C.G. *The Archetypes and the Collective Unconscious.*

Jung, C.G. *Word and Image.*

O'Donohue, John. *Anam Cara: Spiritual Wisdom from the Celtic World.*

O'Donohue, John. *Benedictus: A Book of Blessings.*

River, Jade. *To Know: A Guide to Women's Magic and Spirituality.*

Sams, Jamie. *Dancing the Dream: The Seven Sacred Paths of Human Transformation.*

Starhawk and Hilary Valentine. *The Twelve Wild Swans: A Journey to the Realm of Magic, Healing and Action.*

van Lommel, Pim. *Consciousness Beyond Life: The Science of Near Death Experience.*

Weller, Francis. *Entering the Healing Ground: Grief, Ritual and the Soul of the World.*

Wikman, Monika. *Pregnant Darkness: Alchemy and the Rebirth of Consciousness.*

Nature and Healing

Blackie, Sharon. *If Women Rose Rooted: A Journey to Authenticity and Belonging.*

Blackie, Sharon. *The Enchanted Life.*

Clarke, JJ. *Voices of the Earth: An Anthology of Ideas and Arguments.*

Eisenstein, Charles. *The More Beautiful World Our Hearts Know is Possible.*

Macy, Joanna and Chris Johnstone. *Active Hope: How to Face the Mess We're in Without Going Crazy.*

Macy, Joanna and Molly Young-Brown. *Coming Back to Life: The Updated Guide to the Work that Reconnects.*

Monbiot, George. *Feral: Rewilding the Land, Sea and Human Life.*

Oliver, Mary. *Wild Geese: Selected Poems.*

Plotkin, Bill. *Nature and the Human Soul: Cultivating Wholeness in a Fragmented World*

Plotkin, Bill. *Soulcraft: Crossing into the Mysteries of Nature and Psyche.*

Ryan-Gerhardt, Ciara. *Integra: Stories of Home and Displacement.*

Starhawk. *Dreaming the Dark.*

Starhawk. *The Spiral Dance: A Rebirth of the Ancient Religion of the Great Goddess.*

Tolle, Eckhart. *A New Earth: Create a Better Life.*

Turner, Toko-Pa. *Belonging: Remembering Ourselves Home.*

FILM

Afflicted (Netflix docuseries)

Femme: Women Healing the World

Emerging Proud

The Goddess Project

Heroin(e)

Sicko (a Michael Moore documentary)

Split (a powerful film by Deborah Kampmeier on Inanna's descent)

Hysteria

Heal

Take Your Pills (Netflix documentary)

Dark States – Heroin Town – a Louis Theroux documentary.

The Ascent of Woman (BBC)

Peckham Health Centre Documentary – tiny.cc/peckham

"My Body Is a Prison of Pain so I Want to Leave It Like a Mystic But I Also Love It & Want It to Matter Politically." Hedva, Johanna. johannahedva.com/hospital.html

YOUTUBE

Depression is a Disease of Civilization: Stephen Ilardi at TEDxEmory

An Overview of Archetypal Vision – Caroline Myss

Why People Don't Heal and How They Can – Caroline Myss

MUSIC MEDICINE

This book was created with the musical medicine of these talented artists played on endless repeat for two and a half years. I would love to share my playlist with you on Spotify – you can find it at tinyurl. com/MedicineWomanLHP

Eleanor Brown. *Meet You There;* "We Will Not Be Lost to These Times", "In the Roots We Are Together" (ALisa's Song). Signed copies of *Meet You There* available from shop.womancraftpublishing.com

The Greatest Showman soundtrack – especially "From Now On" and "This is Me" (the live YouTube rehearsal videos)

Medicine for the People. *Dark as Night.*

Rising Appalachia. *Wider Circles; Scale Down; Filthy Dirty South.*

Jennifer Berezan. "Returning"

Xavier Rudd. "Spirit Bird"

GAMES

For those of us who are sick, spend a lot of time in waiting rooms, in bed, unable to read or focus, computer games and virtual reality experiences, available on a phone or tablet, can be an enjoyable way to pass time, and potentially promote healing.

Monument Valley – my all-time favourite, with beautiful scenery based on M. C. Escher's work, soothing music, and practical experience in problem solving and changing perspectives.

ONLINE RESOURCES

Automunity and Chronic Illness

Abbott, Isabel. "Believing the Body". www.isabelabbott.com/writing/2016/9/13/believing-the-body

Gale, E.A.M. "The Epidemiology of Type One Diabetes", Diapedia. www.diapedia.org/type-1-diabetes-mellitus/2104085168/epidemiology-of-type-1-diabetes

Hedva, Johanna. "The Sick Woman Theory", Mask Magazine. www.maskmagazine.com/not-again/struggle/sick-woman-theory

Hopkins, Tamsin. "But You Don't Look Sick". www.ecofluffymama.com/2016/09/dont-look-sick/

Kennedy, Stephanie. "When You're Not Sick Enough". www.butyoudontlooksick.com/articles/personal-essays/when-youre-not-sick-enough

Lazard, Carolyn. "How to Be a Person in the Age of Autoimmunity", The Cluster Mag. theclustermag.com/2013/01/how-to-be-a-person-in-the-age-of-autoimmunity

Leontiades, Louisa. "But I Can Cook". louisaleontiades.com/but-i-can-cook

Mendel, Karon. "When I'm Asked 'What Do You Do?' as a Woman With a Chronic Illness", The Mighty. themighty.com/2016/05/how-to-answer-what-do-you-do-as-a-woman-with-rheumatoid-arthritis

Miserandino, Christine. "The Spoon Theory", www.butyoudontlooksick.com/articles/written-by-christine/the-spoon-theory

O'Rourke, Meghan. "What's Wrong with Me?", New Yorker Magazine. www.newyorker.com/magazine/2013/08/26/whats-wrong-with-me

Weiss, Suzannah. "How Doctors Gaslight Women into Doubting Their Own Pain", Broadly. broadly.vice.com/en_us/article/gy899x/maya-dusenbery-how-doctors-gaslight-women-doubting-their-own-pain

Windling, Terri. "Illness as Narrative". www.terriwindling.com/blog/2016/04/illness-as-narrative.html

Wollen, Audrey. "Sad Girl Theory", Cultist Zine. www.cultistzine.com/2014/06/19/cult-talk-audrey-wollen-on-sad-girl-theory

Wyant, Paige. "28 Signs You Grew Up With an Autoimmune Disease", The Mighty. themighty.com/2018/02/signs-growing-up-with-autoimmune-disease

Social Criticism

Arabi, Shahida. "Why the Women Society Calls 'Damaged' are the Most Powerful". badwitch.es/women-society-calls-damaged-powerful

Brewer, Joe. "The Pain You Feel is Capitalism Dying", Medium.com. medium.com/@joe_brewer/the-pain-you-feel-is-capitalism-dying-5cdbe06a936c

Carrington, Damian. "Rising temperatures linked to increased suicide rates", The Guardian. www.theguardian.com/environment/2018/jul/23/rising-temperatures-linked-to-increased-suicide-rates

Dashu, Max. "Raising the Dead: Medicine Women Who Revive and Retrieve Souls". www.sourcememory.net/veleda/?p=628

Haque, Umair. "Why Our Societies Need Healing." eand.co/why-our-societies-need-healing-f1940dd5c582

Haque, Umair. "Why We're Underestimating the American Collapse". eand.co/why-were-underestimating-american-collapse-be04d9e55235

Hartman, Robert. "Ending Patriarchy", Kindred. kindredmedia.org/2018/06/ending-patriarchy

Jones, Amy. "The Goopification of self-care misrepresents how hard looking after yourself can be", The Pool. www.the-pool.com/health/mind/2018/7/amy-jones-on-the-goopification-of-self-care

Livingston, James. "Fuck Work". aeon.co/essays/what-if-jobs-are-not-the-solution-but-the-problem

Noe Pagán, Camille. "When Doctors Downplay Women's Health Concerns", New York Times. www.nytimes.com/2018/05/03/well/live/when-doctors-downplay-womens-health-concerns.html

Plett, Heather. "This Body, Without the Triumphant Narrative". heatherplett.com/2017/06/body-without-triumphant-narrative

Safi, Omid. "The Disease of Being Busy". onbeing.org/blog/the-disease-of-being-busy

Medicine and Health Care

D'Anconna, Matthew. "From Andrew Wakefield to Brexiteers, snake-oil salesmen are keeping us sick", The Guardian. www.theguardian.com/commentisfree/2018/jul/22/snake-oil-medicine-politics-andrew-wakefield

Devlin, Hannah. "Top oncologist to study effect of diet on cancer drugs", The Guardian. www.theguardian.com/science/2018/jul/06/top-oncologist-to-study-effect-of-diet-on-cancer-drugs

Dossey, Dr. Larry. "Healing Research: What We Know and Don't Know", Explore: The Journal of Science and Healing. www.explorejournal.com/article/S1550-8307(08)00285-1/fulltext

Dossey, Dr. Larry. "Spirituality, Healing and Science", Huffington Post. www.huffingtonpost.com/dr-larry-dossey/spirituality-healing-and_b_680472.html

Dumas, Firoozeh. "After Surgery in Germany, I Wanted Vicodin, Not Herbal Tea", New York Times. www.nytimes.com/2018/01/27/opinion/sunday/surgery-germany-vicodin.html

Fassler, Joe. "How Doctors Take Women's Pain Less Seriously", The Atlantic. www.theatlantic.com/health/archive/2015/10/emergency-room-wait-times-sexism/410515

Hart, Anna. "I'm an adult woman with dyspraxia – realising that changed my life", The Pool. www.the-pool.com/health/health/2018/26/Anna-Hart-on-getting-a-dyspraxia-diagnosis-as-adult-woman

Howick, J. "How empathic is your healthcare practitioner? A systematic review and meta-analysis of patient surveys", BMC Medical Education. bmcmededuc.biomedcentral.com/articles/10.1186/s12909-017-0967-3

Jamison, Leslie. "Grand Unified Theory of Female Pain", VQR. www.vqronline.org/essays-articles/2014/04/grand-unified-theory-female-pain

Larkin, Marilynn. "Pay gaps persist for female and African American physicians in US", Reuters. www.reuters.com/article/us-health-physicians-pay-gaps/pay-gaps-persist-for-female-and-african-american-physicians-in-us-idUSKBN-1HI1E0

Lickerman, Alex. "How emotional trauma often manifests as physical symptoms", Psychology Today. www.psychologytoday.com/us/blog/happiness-in-world/201003/psychosomatic-symptoms

Maté, Gabor. "How to Build a Culture of Good Health", YES! Magazine. www.yesmagazine.org/issues/good-health/gabor-mate-how-to-build-a-culture-of-good-health-20151116

O' Mahony, Claire. "Is Dr Fionnula McHale the future of medical care?" The Independent. www.independent.ie/life/health-wellbeing/is-dr-fionnula-mchale-the-future-of-medical-care-i-make-healthy-people-healthier-with-functional-medicine-31168341.html

Siddique, Haroon. "Women feel patronised by doctors, health minister says." www.theguardian.com/society/2018/jun/29/women-often-feel-patronised-by-doctors-health-minister-says

World Health Organization. www.who.int/mental_health/media/en/242.pdf?ua=1

World Health Organization. www.who.int/mental_health/prevention/genderwomen/en

Mental Health

Andrews, Tracy A. "What is Dissociation Anyway?" healingfromthefreeze.wordpress.com/2011/04/26/what-is-dissociation-anyway

Beck, Martha. "Creativity Tips from Martha". marthabeck.com/2010/10/creativity-tips-from-martha/

Bell, Andrea L. "Why Self-Regulation is the Most Important Thing in the World". www.goodtherapy.org/blog/why-self-regulation-is-most-important-thing-in-world-0807175

Bentall, Professor Richard. "All in the Brain". blogs.canterbury.ac.uk/discursive/all-in-the-brain

Brampton, Sally. "I told myself – 'Get over yourself. Stop snivelling. Stop whining…'", The Telegraph. www.telegraph.co.uk/women/life/sally-brampton-i-told-myself---get-over-yourself-stop-snivelling

Brogan, Kelly. "An Open Letter to the Spiritual Community About Psychiatry". kellybroganmd.com/an-open-letter-to-the-spiritual-community-about-psychiatry

Carrington. Damian. "Air pollution linked to increased mental illness in children", The Guardian. www.theguardian.com/environment/2016/jun/13/air-pollution-linked-to-increased-mental-illness-in-children

Eisenstein, Charles. "Mutiny of the Soul Revisited". newandancientstory.net/mutiny-of-the-soul-revisited

Eisenstein, Charles. "Mutiny of the Soul". charleseisenstein.net/mutiny

Gordon, James S. "Drugs alone won't fix our epidemic of depression", The Guardian. www.theguardian.com/society/commentisfree/2018/jul/19/drugs-alone-wont-fix-our-epidemic-of-depression

Hari, Johann. "Is Everything You Know About Depression Wrong?", The Guardian. www.theguardian.com/society/2018/jan/07/is-everything-you-think-you-know-about-depression-wrong-johann-hari-lost-connections

Hulk. "Antony Bourdain, Suicide and Grace", The Observer. observer.com/2018/06/anthony-bourdain-suicide-and-grace

Lawrence, Tim. "Everything Doesn't Happen for a Reason". www.timjlawrence.com/blog/2015/10/19/everything-doesnt-happen-for-a-reason

Malcolm, Lynne and Prof Peter Kinderman. "Does mental 'illness' exist?" All in the Mind, RN. www.abc.net.au/radionational/programs/allinthemind/does-mental-illness-exist/9130774

Morgan, Eleanor. "Female Hysteria and Metal Health", The Pool. www.the-pool.com/health/mind/2016/23/eleanor-morgan-on-female-hysteria-and-mental-health

Nerenberg, Jenara. "Why Neurodiversity Matters in Health Care", Aspen Institute. www.aspeninstitute.org/blog-posts/neurodiversity-matters-health-care

Rosenberg, Robin. "Abnormal is the New Normal", Slate. www.slate.com/articles/health_and_science/medical_examiner/2013/04/diagnostic_and_statistical_manual_fifth_edition_why_will_half_the_u_s_population.html

Sarkis, Stephanie A. "11 Warning Signs of Gaslighting", Psychology Today. www.psychologytoday.com/us/blog/here-there-and-everywhere/201701/11-warning-signs-gaslighting

Webster, Bethany. "Releasing the Need to Struggle". www.wombofflight.com/releasing-the-need-to-struggle/

Statistics

www.ons.gov.uk

www.cdc.gov

stats.oecd.org

www.cwhn.ca

www.womenshealth.gov

www.ncbi.nlm.nih.gov

www.aarda.org

who.int

www.health.org.uk

sgwhc.org

www.nhs.uk

minoritynurse.com/nursing-statistics

www.theguardian.com/healthcare-network/2017/mar/01/why-so-few-male-nurses

en.wikipedia.org/wiki/Women_in_medicine

www.nhsemployers.org/~/media/Employers/Publications/Gender%20in%20the%20NHS

www.midwife.org/Essential-Facts-about-Midwives

www.ted.com/talks/alyson_mcgregor_why_medicine_often_has_dangerous_side_effects_for_women

WEBSITES

Neurodiversity, Asperger's and Autism in Women

autismawarenesscentre.com

www.aane.org

autismwomensnetwork.org

avoicereleased.co.uk

www.facebook.com/intunepathways

spectrumnews.com

Jenara Nerenberg & The Neurodiversity Project

Mental Health – Positive Approaches

The Artidote – on Facebook

Mad in America

The Icarus Project – website, on the ground and on Facebook

Sanctuary for Terror – on Facebook

The Fluent Self

Emerging Proud – Film on mental illness and spiritual transformation. Watch online emergingproud.com

Chronic Health Conditions and Healing

themighty.com

theunchargeables.com

womenswellnesscircle.lpages.co

www.activehope.info

www.hfme.org

wearecanaries.com

myheartsisters.org

workthatreconnects.org

www.rccxandillness.com

www.aarda.org

www.paulayoumellrn.com

Women's Health

www.brighamandwomens.org/research

www.laurabushinstitute.org

www.womenshealth.gov

www.cwhn.ca

whri.org

INDEX

ABOUT THE AUTHOR

LUCY H. PEARCE is the author of numerous life-changing non-fiction books for women and a vibrant artist of lost archetypes of the feminine and spiral forms.

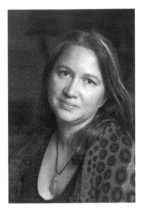

Several of her books have been Amazon #1 bestsellers around the world, including the Nautilus silver-award-winning *Burning Woman* – an incendiary exploration of women and power – written for every woman who burns with passion, has been burned with shame, and in another time or place would be burned at the stake; *The Rainbow Way: cultivating creativity in the midst of motherhood* and *Moon Time: harness the ever-changing energy of your menstrual cycle*.

An award-winning, first-class graduate of Kingston University with a BA in History of Ideas and English Literature, and teaching graduate of Trinity College, Cambridge, Lucy's work is dedicated to supporting women's creative, empowered, embodied expression through her writing, teaching and art. Her writing – spanning from pregnancy and birth, parenting, women's health and creativity – has appeared internationally in mainstream and alternative publications. She is a regular speaker and guest teacher on online events.

A mother of three, she lives on the coast in East Cork, Ireland, where she runs Womancraft Publishing – creating life-changing, paradigm-shifting books by women, for women – with her husband.

You can find an archive of her blogs, interviews and articles, discover upcoming opportunities to learn with Lucy, and subscribe to her newsletter at: www.lucyhpearce.com

ABOUT THE COVER ARTIST

HÜLYA ÖZDEMIR is an illustrator and painter of watercolour portraits. Born in Istanbul in 1972, she has been living in Bodrum in the South Aegean for three years.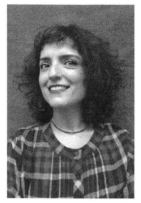

One of the 'The Printemps des Artistes' (The Spring of the Artists) artists, she has had two solo exhibitions and participated in two group exhibitions for charity. Her art has appeared on magazines and books around the world.

Although she focuses on predominantly female portraits, she does not set any restrictions on her drawings. What guides her is the understanding that a woman is a person who still struggles to exist in a male-dominated society, imprisoned in a role based on maintaining norms of society: tradition, morality, and family triangles, as an asset whose desires, vulnerabilities and worries often do not reflect her own feelings. In her artwork we see women becoming increasingly self-confident, re-establishing their human identity, as the artist enriches the exposition of these inner worlds with patterns.

WOMANCRAFT PUBLISHING

Womancraft Publishing was founded on the revolutionary vision that women and words can change the world. We act as midwife to transformational women's words that have the power to challenge, inspire, heal and speak to the silenced aspects of ourselves.

We believe that:

- ◑ books are a fabulous way of transmitting powerful transformation,

- ◑ values should be juicy actions, lived out,

- ◑ ethical business is a key way to contribute to conscious change.

At the heart of our Womancraft philosophy is fairness and integrity. Creatives and women have always been underpaid. Not on our watch! We split royalties 50:50 with our authors. We work on a full circle model of giving and receiving: reaching backwards, supporting TreeSisters' reforestation projects, and forwards via Worldreader, providing books at no-cost to education projects for girls and women.

We are proud that Womancraft is walking its talk and engaging so many women each year via our books and online. Join the revolution! Sign up to the mailing list at womancraftpublishing.com and find us on social media for exclusive offers:

- ⓕ womancraftpublishing
- ⓨ womancraftbooks
- ⓘ womancraft_publishing

If you loved this book, and want to help spread the Womancraft message, you can!

- ① *post a short review*
- ① *tell your friends about it*
- ① *share it on social media*

YOU ARE INVITED TO JOIN LUCY
AND THE COMMUNITY OF WOMEN
READING THIS BOOK ON THE
"MEDICINE WOMAN – A BOOK BY LUCY H. PEARCE"
FACEBOOK GROUP.

ALSO FROM WOMANCRAFT PUBLISHING

BURNING WOMAN
Lucy H. Pearce

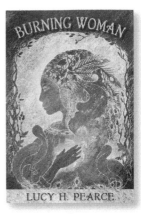

A breath-taking and controversial woman's journey through history - personal and cultural - on a quest to find and free her own power.

Uncompromising and all-encompassing, Pearce uncovers the archetype of the Burning Women of days gone by - Joan of Arc and the witch trials, through to the way women are burned today in cyber bullying, acid attacks, shaming and burnout, fearlessly examining the roots of Feminine power - what it is, how it has been controlled, and why it needs to be unleashed on the world in our modern Burning Times.

A must-read for all women! A life-changing book that fills the reader with a burning passion and desire for change.

Glennie Kindred, author of Earth Wisdom

MOON TIME: HARNESS THE EVER-CHANGING ENERGY OF YOUR MENSTRUAL CYCLE
Lucy H. Pearce

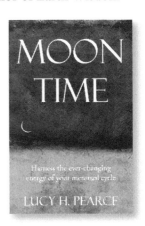

Hailed as 'life-changing' by women around the world, *Moon Time* shares a fully embodied understanding of the menstrual cycle. Full of practical insight, empowering resources, creative activities and passion, this book will put women back in touch with their body's wisdom.

Lucy, your book is monumental. The wisdom in Moon Time sets a new course where we glimpse a future culture reshaped by honoring our womanhood journeys one woman at a time.

ALisa Starkweather, founder of the Red Tent Temple Movement

FULL CIRCLE HEALTH: INTEGRATED HEALTH CHARTING FOR WOMEN

Lucy H. Pearce

Welcome to *Full Circle Health*. A creative approach to holistic health for all who love planners, trackers and bullet journals to guide and support you in a greater understanding of your physical, mental and emotional health.

Whether menstruating or not, pregnant or post-partum, *Full Circle Health* provides a highly flexible, deeply supportive way of tracking your health, whatever your current health conditions.

WILD & WISE: SACRED FEMININE MEDITATIONS FOR WOMEN'S CIRCLES AND PERSONAL AWAKENING

Amy Bammel Wilding

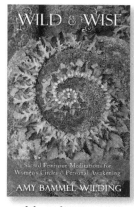

The stunning debut by Amy Bammel Wilding is not merely a collection of guided meditations, but a potent tool for personal and global transformation. The meditations beckon you to explore the powerful realm of symbolism and archetypes, inviting you to access your wild and wise inner knowing.

Suitable for reflective reading or to facilitate healing and empowerment for women who gather in red tents, moon lodges, women's circles and ceremonies.

This rich resource is an answer to "what can we do to go deeper?" that many in circles want to know.

Jean Shinoda Bolen, MD

Printed in Great Britain
by Amazon